SEXUAL IDEOLOGY *and* SCHOOLING

SEXUAL IDEOLOGY
and SCHOOLING

Towards Democratic Sexuality Education

Alexander McKay

State University of New York Press

First published in U.S.A. in 1999 by
State University of New York Press
Albany

For information, address State University of New York Press,
State University Plaza, Albany, NY 12246

Printed in Canada

Library of Congress Cataloging-in-Publication Data

McKay, Alexander, 1962-
Sexual ideology and schooling : towards democratic sexuality education / Alexander McKay.
p.   cm.
Includes bibliographical references (p.) and index.
ISBN 0-7914-4523-2 (hard : alk. paper). — ISBN 0-7914-4524-0 (pbk. : alk. paper)
1. Sex instruction for children. 2. Sex instruction for youth. 3. Politics and education. 4. Sexual ethics—Study and teaching. I. Title.
HQ57.3.M35   1999
613.9'07—dc21
99-37849
CIP

10 9 8 7 6 5 4 3 2 1

For Ella McKay
1889-1977

Table of Contents

Preface

—··—··—

As anyone who has even dabbled in the subject knows, the study of sexuality education in the schools extends far beyond the standard principles of classroom teaching and learning. Uncovering the dynamics that set the course of sexuality education requires much more than an investigation into pedagogical theory. First and foremost, we are compelled, by necessity, to begin by examining the wider social, moral, and political contexts in which sexuality education takes place. As this book makes clear, the public and academic discourse on sexuality education in the schools is, at its essence, a conversation, usually a highly argumentative one, between competing perspectives on sexual politics and morality. This is worthy of consideration not only because of its ramifications for what goes on in the sexuality education classroom, but also because the discourse around, and practice of, sexuality education provides an illuminating and instructive guide to understanding the contemporary debates about sexuality in Western culture.

Among the most important functions of education is to prepare young people to become active participants in society. Jerome Bruner (1996) looks at education as a "test frame" for our ideas about cultural psychology. Culture is the toolkit through which we construct our world and define who we are. The shape and course of education, then, can only be properly understood in terms of its cultural context. How we educate youth to absorb and employ the cultural toolkit, as part of facilitating their development as human beings, speaks volumes about our vision of society. It is through education that we learn the skills, social norms, and values that allow us to successfully integrate into society, giving us the potential to lead fulfilling and productive lives. It is also by way of education that we learn of our rights and obligations as citizens of a democracy.

Looking at the educational process from this perspective suggests that sexuality education involves facilitating young people's ability to develop and maintain a healthy, satisfying, and morally responsible sexuality. But what is a healthy, satisfying, and morally responsible sexuality? The conflict over the answer to this question preoccupies our culture. The issues that come to the foreground in deciding the shape and content of sexuality education in the schools are at the very centre of the divisive conflict over sexuality taking place in our society. Many of the points of debate around sexual orientation, childhood sexuality, adolescent childbearing, the link between love and sex, gender relations, contraception, and the role of sexuality in maintaining the nuclear family as a social/economic structure become flash points in the discussion of what public institutions such as the school should be teaching young people about sexuality. Because of its role in moulding us as individuals and social actors, education may be an ideal template for exploring reasonable and democratic approaches to sexuality in our society.

As I will document in this book, a lot rides on sexuality with respect to its implications for the moral and social make up of Western society. Whether or not our collective culture comes to first accept and then affirm moral and behavioural diversity in sexual norms and practices will be one of the most important developments to shape the fabric of Western society in the 21st century. My initial and primary purpose in writing this book is to illustrate how sexuality education in the schools has been suffocated by the influence of ideology, and to articulate the parameters of a better and more just sexuality education that corresponds to the ideals of a democratic society. By extension, however, this book conceives of sexuality education as an apt "test frame" for how we, as a democratic culture, can begin looking at sexuality not from the often rigid tunnel vision of sexual ideologies but from a broader perspective more closely aligned to the moral, social, and political ideals of the democratic tradition. The ideological debates around sexuality education in the schools are the wider social and moral conflicts related to sexuality in our culture writ large.

Acknowledgements

- . — . — . — . — .

A number of people have contributed to the development of the ideas expressed in this book. In particular, I wish to thank Gerald McKay, Michael Barrett, Ronald Morris and William Lawlor. Their insights on human sexuality and sexuality education have influenced me considerably. I am especially grateful to Dwight Boyd, my thesis supervisor at the Ontario Institute for Studies in Education/University of Toronto for his guidance, challenging questions, excellent suggestions for further reading, and constructive comments on earlier drafts of the manuscript. Thanks to The Althouse Press team for their enthusiasm, editorial skills, and guidance during the publication process. The library of the Sex Information and Education Council of Canada (SIECCAN) was an invaluable source of information and research.

Introduction

—··—··——··—

Sexuality education in the schools is not a new idea. Since the late 19th century, schools have played an active role in helping young people learn about human sexuality (Bruess & Greenberg, 1994). For example, in 1905, the American Society for Sanitary and Moral Prophylaxis began conducting classes in the schools on sexually transmitted diseases. "They called for a return to Victorian values, emphasizing the 'pure' nature of women and the importance of sexual restraint in men" (Strong & Devault, 1994, p. 216). During the early part of the 20th century, social hygienists in Canada were using the concept of nature study to introduce sexuality education in the schools with the hope that children would "understand the basics of reproduction without having their sexual instincts prematurely aroused, and be able to steel themselves with this knowledge when faced with the possibility of sexual corruption in word or deed" (Sethna, 1994, p. 192). By the early 1990s, nearly every state in the United States and every province in Canada either mandated or strongly recommended that some form of sexuality education be provided in the schools.

From its inception, however, sexuality education in the schools has been a highly controversial issue. As the comprehensiveness and explicitness of sexuality education has increased, the controversies surrounding it have become more volatile and frequent. Pitched battles over the objectives and nature of school-based sexuality education are increasingly occurring in communities across North America (Rienzo, 1989; Kantor, 1994; Sedway, 1992; Ross & Kantor, 1995). One of the results of these controversies is that sexuality education in the schools has been unable to reach its full potential in helping young people protect and enhance their sexual health. For example, as Ehrhardt, Yingling, and Warne (1991) suggest,

1

sex education programs in the United States have been troubled by controversy over whether schools and parents should encourage abstinence as a "moral stance" or should accept sexuality as an important marker of adolescent development and develop realistic educational programs. Because of the absence of a clear message that takes into account the realities of adolescent sexuality, this country has not been as successful as other Western countries in preventing unwanted teenage pregnancies. Similarly, the effectiveness of educational programs to prevent HIV/AIDS and other STDs has been severely hampered by debates of morality, taste, and religion rather than a realistic public health approach. (p. 36)

Tragically, these kinds of moral disputes, particularly in the United States, have constrained the ability of educators to provide effective AIDS prevention education programs. Anke Ehrhardt (1996) of the HIV Center for Clinical and Behavioral Studies at Columbia University astutely observes "The debate is fueled by strong beliefs and convictions of right and wrong and leaves little room for an impartial assessment of the facts and a definition of pragmatic goals" (p. 1524).

A study conducted by The Alan Guttmacher Institute found that "teachers regard pressure from parents, the community or school administration as the major problem they face in providing sexuality education" (Forrest & Silverman, 1989, p. 65). Earls, Fraser and Sumpter (1992) state that "When it comes to public education, the sexuality curriculum is mired in conflicting influences" (p. 200) and Bruess and Greenberg (1994) note that "In the 1990s there has been a growing wave of censorship ravaging sexuality education in communities and states around the nation" (p. 58).

These comments help to show that sexuality education is, without question, one of the most controversial subjects ever to be introduced into the public school. While there are frequent disagreements about the best way to teach reading, writing and arithmetic, these disputes do not typically involve considerations of morality, taste, and religion. Although the teaching of history, English literature and other so called "social studies" has been prone to controversy along lines similar to that of sexuality education, seldom have these quarrels reached the same intensity as the battles over the appropriate nature and content of instruction in human sexuality. Relevant, meaningful, and effective sexuality education in the schools is unlikely to occur unless we can establish a framework to mediate these quarrels.

Some of the conflicts surrounding sexuality education in the schools appear irresolvable. Our beliefs about the nature and purpose of human sexuality are often very strongly held and they dictate, to a great extent, what we believe should be taught in the sexuality education classroom. For example our society is clearly divided on the issue of homosexuality. Some people believe that homosexual behaviour is wrong, while others believe it is acceptable. As a result, some people believe strongly that sexuality education should teach young people that homosexuality is immoral as well as psychologically and socially dysfunctional, while other people feel just as strongly that young people should be taught that homosexuality can be both morally acceptable and healthy.

Many people feel that the existing structure of social norms related to sexuality contributes to inequality between the sexes, while others believe that "traditional" gender arrangements represent natural differences between men and women that should not be disturbed. Consequently, some people believe sexuality education in the schools should teach young people to rebel against traditional gender arrangements, while others believe that sexuality education should reflect what are held to be the innate differences between male and female sexuality. Some people strongly believe that premarital sex is immoral and unacceptably dangerous for the health of young people, while others believe that sexual relations between unmarried people is acceptable provided that the participants mutually consent to the activity and that health precautions are taken. In turn, some people believe that with respect to premarital sex, sexuality education in the schools should focus exclusively on promoting premarital sexual abstinence, while others believe that in addition to discussing abstinence, sexuality education should provide young people with contraceptive and safer sex information. These conflicts of perspective are played out in the ongoing debates about sexuality education in the schools. They suggest that our opinions about the form and content of sexuality education are, as we might expect, strongly tied to our moral convictions about human sexuality.

Schools are increasingly being called upon to provide sexuality education. Yet, because public perspectives toward sexuality education are so imbued by often deeply held moral values related to some of the most critical and hotly contested social issues of our time, educators find themselves confronting immensely challenging pedagogical questions. Will youth be taught to embrace the values of chastity, monogamy, and the nuclear family model of sexuality? Will they be taught to see procreation or intimacy or recreation as the primary purpose of sexuality? Will they be taught to accept the moral legitimacy of homosexuality? Will they be encouraged to critically evaluate prevailing social constructions of gender? Will their sexuality education programs be based on religious or secular conceptualizations of human sexuality?

Educators caught in the glare of sexuality education controversies are being asked, if not compelled, to provide answers to these highly sensitive questions. If these answers are not persuasive enough to satisfy competing community interests, the development of effective and meaningful school-based programs comes to an abrupt halt. In my work with the Sex Information and Education Council of Canada (SIECCAN), I have frequently acted as a consultant for school boards and public health departments grappling with these questions. My experience strongly suggests that credible responses to these often vexing queries about the nature and content of sexuality education requires that educators think carefully about the philosophical foundations of the programs they hope to teach, something few sexuality educators are trained to do.

My experience in this field leads me to conclude that many educators involved in providing sexuality education in the public schools understand the importance of this topic and are committed to providing sexuality education that, as much as possible, meets the often diverse educational needs of their students. While none of us can fully escape our own values when teaching young people about sexuality, most sexuality educators seek to be relatively nonjudgemental and unbiased in their teaching. They want students to think critically about sexuality, making informed decisions about this critical aspect of their lives. In the face of pervasive conflict over sexual norms and values in our society, how can sexuality educators articulate and defend a philosophy of sexuality education that is aimed at helping young people arrive at fully informed, critically appropriated choices?

My goal in writing this book is to travel through the intellectual minefield of perplexing issues and questions that educators must ultimately address head-on if they are to constructively contribute to the young people's right to a democratic sexuality education. Thus, this book is primarily aimed at educators and all those concerned with providing high quality sexuality education in the schools. I have made an attempt to contextualize and explore these issues and questions with more background and intellectual depth than is commonly the case in the contemporary discourse on sexuality education in the schools. The failure of current sexuality education debates to be adequately resolved to the point where meaningful school-based programs become possible is the result of a lack of rigorous analysis and dialogue related to the most fundamental questions about the nature of sexuality, its role in shaping our society, and most importantly of all, how differences of moral perspective toward sexuality ought to be accommodated in a democratic society. To fully address these questions takes us beyond the sphere of education and thrusts us into the realms of moral philosophy, philosophy of science, sociology, history, and sexology. As such, I hope this book will be of interest not only to sexuality educators but also to those interested in the philosophy and sociology of human sexuality, particularly as they relate to public policy issues.

Many of us who work in professions related to sexual health are sometimes troubled by, or directly confronted with, the lack of a clear coherent philosophical grounding for our work. Whether we are educators, clinicians, therapists, or academic sexologists, we are, hopefully, well equipped with the skills and methodologies to conduct our work effectively. Nevertheless, we are frequently hampered by the lack of a philosophical framework with which to justify and explain our work, particularly to those who do not approve of the way we do it or would prefer that we did not do it at all. Sexologists from a variety of disciplines can make an important positive contribution to our society, but it will not be good enough, for reasons that will become clear in this book, for us to simply come forth to propose ever more advanced theories and practices, no matter how obviously beneficial to us they appear, unless we have a clear and highly credible philosophy that enables us to explain and defend what we do. This book attempts to create such a philosophy with respect to sexuality education, the subdiscipline of sexology within which I do most of my work. It is my hope, however, that the philosophy of sexuality education presented in these pages will be useful and relevant to my colleagues in other subdisciplines of sexology whose work is invariably affected by the ongoing conflicts of sexual ideology in our culture.

The emphasis on key democratic principles, which serves as the foundation of this philosophy, is not intended to function simply as a defensive shield against those who question our motives or oppose the enterprise of sexual health promotion. Just as importantly, a democratic philosophy of sexuality education is only really democratic when it functions to help those who create and implement curricula, conduct sexological research, provide therapy and counselling, advocate for high quality sexuality education and clinical services, and those who make public policy decisions to reflect upon their own biases and assumptions. It is only with critical reflection upon our own perspectives that we can make the necessary modifications to ensure that our work is indeed consistent with the principles of democracy. If we are armed with this critical self-reflection, a devotion to democratic principles, and a credible philosophical framework to justify and explain what we are doing, sexuality educators and others in professional fields related to sexuality will be more capable of seeing that the roadblocks that have hampered our ability to make important contributions to the community are gradually removed.

Over the course of this book I will examine the fundamental issues relevant to the development of a philosophy of sexuality education in the schools that is appropriate for a democratic society where profound differences of opinion and moral conviction related to human sexuality exist. At its essence, a democratic philosophy of sexuality education must accomplish two primary tasks. First, it must find a way to acknowledge and respect moral pluralism related to sexuality. Respect for moral pluralism is a fundamental tenet of democratic society. Second, a democratic philosophy of sexuality education must not only respect the differing moral perspectives toward sexuality that exist in society, but it must also foster the democratic right of all people, including young people, to deliberate between different points of view in arriving at their own convictions. This, too, is a fundamental tenet of democratic society. Both of these tasks, I believe, logically lead us to a focus on the most fundamental of all democratic rights: Freedom of belief. A democratic philosophy of sexuality education must respect and promote freedom of belief.

Given the nature of prevailing differences of moral perspectives related to human sexuality that characterize contemporary Western society, and given the nature of the debates around sexuality education in the schools, articulating a philosophy of sexuality education founded on the democratic right of freedom of belief raises a number of complex and perplexing issues. We need to deepen our understanding of the debate about sexuality education.

The first step in understanding the conflict over sexuality education in the schools is to discern why this issue is so passionately fought over. Why is sexuality education so controversial? In Chapter One, I suggest that sexuality education is the site of intense conflict because it is a key battle ground in a wider debate about the nature of society itself. What we teach young people about human sexuality will at least partially influence the shape of society's future social norms. Social norms related to sexuality are widely regarded as being an important determinant of the nature of society and we are deeply divided as a culture as to the appropriate shape and substance of these norms. Thus, we cannot accurately understand the sexuality education debates until we see them in terms of the wider ideological disputes related to sexuality that exist in Western culture.

In Chapter Two, I provide an analytical framework for clarifying the conflicts around human sexuality that permeate Western culture. These conflicts are, first and foremost, conflicts of ideology. That is, our society's disagreements related to sexuality are not trivial differences of opinion but rather represent a clash of opposing systems of belief about the nature of the world and humankind. Our ideologies help us to answer fundamental questions about ourselves and the world we live in. In other words, they help us to define and frame reality. The Western cultural discourse on sexuality can be categorized as a struggle between what I call the Restrictive and Permissive sexual ideologies. The Restrictive and Permissive sexual ideologies consist of diametrically opposed, yet internally consistent, beliefs about the nature and purpose of sexuality in human life and society. Although this classification of sexual ideology is quite broad, I will, through a descriptive analysis, show that the conceptual distinctions between Restrictive and Permissive sexual ideology accurately represent the conflict over sexuality in Western culture. Thus, an analysis of the philosophical presuppositions underlying these sexual ideologies is an important step in uncovering the nature of the sexuality education debates. Not surprisingly, the proponents of the Restrictive and Permissive sexual ideologies have very different views on the form and content of sexuality education in the schools.

In Chapter Three, I apply the categories of Restrictive and Permissive sexual ideology to an analysis of sexuality education in the schools. Specifically, I examine the manner and degree to which the presuppositions underlying the Restrictive and Permissive sexual ideologies have influenced the form and content of sexuality education in the schools. This influence has taken several forms. In some cases, sexuality education programs are derived almost entirely from either Restrictive or Permissive sexual ideology. In other cases, sexuality education consists of a conflicting melange of ideological premises regarding human sexuality. In still other cases, the enduring conflict between the Restrictive and Permissive sexual ideologies has cast an aura of controversy around sexuality education in the schools, and as a result educational programs are reduced, as a matter of political expediency, to the provision of an absolute minimum of information and skills related to human sexuality. These "bare-bones" programs are common and they are very often superfluous and irrelevant to students' educational needs. Examining sexuality education in the schools in terms of the influence of sexual ideology on the form and content of educational programs suggests that, among other things, in many cases sexuality education in the schools functions as an instrument of ideological indoctrination rather than as an educational forum for critical deliberation and intellectual development.

In essence, the debate over the form and content of sexuality education in the schools has been focussed on the issue of which set of ideological presuppositions ought to inform educational practice. The firm believers of both the Restrictive and Permissive sexual ideologies assume that truth is on their side. Because they are armed with *the truth*, the proponents of each ideology may feel justified in insisting that their ideological presuppositions related to sexuality become the basis for sexuality education in the schools. But is it really possible to arrive at a genuinely authentic or definitively objective conclusion regarding the true nature and purpose of human sexuality? With respect to the current debate on sexuality education, how we answer this question has significant implications for determining the appropriate objectives of educational programs.

In Chapter Four, I employ a social constructionist analysis of human sexuality to argue that arriving at *the truth* about sexuality in either a scientific or philosophical sense is inescapably dependent on our presuppositional lenses for perceiving the reality of how the world operates. These presuppositional lenses are social constructs rather than precise representations of objective reality. A social constructionist analysis of human sexuality strongly suggests that truth claims about the nature and purpose of human sexuality are seldom immune to legitimate critique. A social constructionist analysis invites us to acknowledge a multiplicity of truths about sexuality. If an epistemological consensus regarding *the truth* about the nature and purpose of sexuality eludes us, the fact of ideological pluralism related to sexuality should, at least in a democratic society, have profound implications for the form and content of sexuality education.

In Chapter Five, I outline the foundational components of a democratic philosophy of sexuality education. Democratic societies are founded, in part, on the principle that moral pluralism is to be both tolerated and respected. This can clearly be seen in the fact that constitutional democracies invariably enshrine the right to freedom of belief as perhaps the most basic element of the cultural or national ethos. Given the fact of the ideological pluralism related to sexuality that characterizes Western culture, the principles of democracy provide an appropriate framework in which to seek ways to accommodate diverse and often opposing perspectives on human sexuality. In exploring further the manner in which a democratic society accommodates and mediates between varied and conflicting belief systems I will use the theory of political liberalism as articulated by philosopher John Rawls. In *Political Liberalism*, Rawls (1993) suggests that democratic societies are characterized by a plurality of religious, philosophical, and moral doctrines. No one of these doctrines is affirmed by all members of society. Furthermore, one doctrine is often incompatible with another. This kind of social-political environment contributes to basic freedoms but cannot guarantee a harmonious relationship between incompatible doctrines. However, what enables democratic societies to persevere, according to Rawls, is that we are bound together, despite our many differences, by our agreement to live by and respect the essentials of a democratic regime. Provided that a particular doctrine does not reject the essentials of a democratic regime, a society based upon the principles of political liberalism has little or nothing to say about the correctness or validity of various religious, philosophical, or moral doctrines. Political liberalism is concerned only with that minimum set of values that define us as a democratic society.

Using the theory of political liberalism as a way of understanding how a democratic society addresses the problem of accommodating incompatible doctrines provides a relevant and applicable foundation for identifying the key features of a democratic philosophy of sexuality education. The debate over the form and content of sexuality education in the schools is a vivid example of the challenge, in free and democratic societies of how to accommodate moral pluralism. Political liberalism suggests, for example, that democratic sexuality education is not based upon judgements about the correctness or superiority of either Restrictive or Permissive sexual ideology. Democratic sexuality education is, however, deeply committed to promoting democratic values. It is committed to the affirmation of moral pluralism and freedom of belief.

In Chapter Six, I explore, in more specific terms, the nature of democratic sexuality education in the schools. In particular, I focus on the need for sexuality education to foster in students the ability to deliberate critically between competing ideological perspectives toward sexuality. Developing this ability in students is important for a number of reasons. For example, critical deliberation contributes to the ability of people to exercise freedom of belief. The process of critical deliberation, of weighing, contrasting, and evaluating differing points of view perpetuates democratic culture. It prepares students for democratic citizenship. In addition, I argue that providing young people with the opportunity to deliberate between differing ideological perspectives toward sexuality increases the likelihood of critical appropriation and genuine attachment to moral convictions related to sexuality.

In Chapter Seven, I discuss, from the standpoint of a democratic philosophy of sexuality education, three of the most controversial issues in the sexuality education debates. There has been considerable debate about how school-based sexuality education should address the issues of sexual orientation, gender equality, and prevention of sexually transmitted diseases and pregnancy. Approaching these issues from a democratic philosophy of sexuality education will represent a fundamental transformation in the way these issues are typically treated in the classroom.

Ultimately, our ideas about what constitutes a good education are tied to our ideas about what constitutes a good society. Formal education presumably plays a key role in preparing people to become active participants in the ongoing development of society. An important litmus test for any philosophy of education is whether or not its principles and practices contribute to this development. In the Conclusion, I discuss the potential of a democratic theory of sexuality education to make a positive contribution to the development of society in general. This discussion is particularly relevant to the perpetual clash between the Restrictive and Permissive sexual ideologies in our culture. Will a democratic form of sexuality education, based on the principles of political liberalism, contribute to a reasonable and just accommodation of moral pluralism related to sexuality in our society? A number of feminist, gay, lesbian and other scholars have quite correctly pointed out that the liberal tradition in Western society has failed to fully deliver on its promise of liberty and equality for all.

Nevertheless, I will argue that the application of the principles of political liberalism to mediate the clash of sexual ideologies in our culture represents a significant and positive transformation of the status quo where social policy related to sexuality is often dictated by ideology rather than democratic principles. Solutions to social strife related to sexuality must inevitably take account of the fact of ideological diversity. Political liberalism seems well suited to this task given its emphasis on accommodating moral pluralism within the boundaries of a democratic culture. Let me be very clear, however, that I am not making claims for the principles of democratic liberalism as universal or entirely objective truths. One critique of liberalism is that it is in fact not neutral, but rather masks its insistence on a particular vision of the good life under the guise of being unbiased and neutral. To the extent that democratic liberalism insists upon, or at least hopes for, citizens who form their values and judgements upon critical deliberation between different points of view, the claim that liberalism is indeed based on particular ideals of the human good is correct. Carmichael (1994) succinctly sums up the gist of the liberal ideal when he writes that "Philosophically, the core commitment of liberalism is a belief in the potential dignity of each individual and in the value of liberty as the essential means of realizing this dignity" (pp. 60-61). I wish neither to refute nor to defend this characteristic of liberalism. But I do want to argue strongly that the basic principles of democratic liberalism constitute the primary ethos of Western culture, and that they have enough broad-based appeal to form the basis upon which we can create a constructive dialogue leading to better and less ideologically laden forms of sexuality education than what is being taught in our schools today.

In discussing the philosophy of sexuality education presented in this book, I have found that it has been generally well received. The idea that sexuality education in the schools ought to be grounded in democratic principles that emphasize the value of relatively unencumbered critical deliberation between what various sexual ideologies have to say about how we should conduct our lives and protect our sexual health makes good sense to most people. However, I am very much aware that there are some people who will object to the philosophy of sexuality education presented in this book.

Among those who will object most strongly are those who cannot tolerate or reconcile themselves to the idea that their own children, or other children for that matter, will be exposed to values and perspectives contrary to their own firmly held sexual ideologies. Democratic concepts such as critical deliberation, respect for different points of view, and freedom of belief, particularly if they are exercised by young people, are subsumed and obliterated by the unbending conviction that any deviation from a particular, and usually very narrow, sexual ideology is not to be tolerated. Those who hold this view believe that public institutions such as the school must be used to inculcate a particular sexual ideology and that alternative perspectives must not be heard. Those who are utterly and irrevocably committed to such a view will have little use for this book. However, those who are more respectful of the moral pluralism that is a fact of our democratic culture, particularly those who have the responsibility for setting educational policy, may find the philosophy of sexuality education set out in the following pages a useful framework for creating and implementing sexuality education in the face of sometimes extreme ideological disagreement. My intention is to provide a justification and rationale for sexuality education programs consistent with the highest and most basic ideals of democracy. Although I do not wish to claim that no examples of democratic sexuality education can be found in our culture, my research and experience in this field leads me to conclude that they are few and far between.

CHAPTER ONE

Sexuality and Sexuality Education: Implications For the Nature of Society

▬ ·· ▬ ·· ▬ ·· ▬ ·· ▬ ·· ▬ ·· ▬ ·· ▬ ·· ▬ ·· ▬ ·· ▬ ·· ▬ ·· ▬ ·

> "...debates about sexuality are debates about the nature of society; as sex goes, so goes society."
>
> (Weeks, 1986)
>
> "Learning a culturally prescribed way of life includes learning sexuality, having the expression of one's sex drive culturally shaped."
>
> (Henslin, 1978)
>
> "Sex education is potentially a vehicle for social engineering par excellence, be it progressive or traditional."
>
> (Thompson, 1994)

Introduction

My objective in this first chapter is to shed some light on why sexuality education in the schools has become so controversial. I propose that the nature of sexuality education is so passionately fought over because, as an instrument in the sexual socialization of youth, sexuality education is seen to play a role in the shaping of sexual values and behavioural norms of our culture which in turn are widely perceived to impact significantly on the character of society as a whole. Sexuality education in the schools is a key battle ground in a wider social conflict about sexuality in particular and the nature of society in general. In other words, the battle over sexuality education is not simply a dispute over the most effective means to promote the sexual and reproductive health of youth, but rather it is, first and foremost, a clash over the shape and direction of society itself. Thus, we can only make sense out of different perspectives on sexuality education in the schools when we consider them in the context of divergent perceptions of the role sexuality should play in promoting a stable and just society.

Sexuality and the Nature Of Society

There is a long held belief that attitudes and values "pertaining to sexual behavior are of the highest importance for both the survival and effectiveness of society" (Kardiner, 1955, p. 23). Indeed, since its very beginning, Western civilization has tended to define itself, in large measure, by its moral, social, and economic organization of human sexuality. As Jeffrey Weeks (1986) puts it, "Concern with sexuality has been at the heart of Western preoccupations since before the triumph of Christianity" (p. 89). The ascension of Christianity as the dominant meaning system of Western society is a key event in the modern history of sexuality, and the importance placed upon sex by the foundational Christian scholars remains with us to this day. Elaine Pagels (1988), in tracing the roots of Christian beliefs about sexuality, suggests that the theologian Augustine (353-430) was the pivotal figure in laying the foundation of the Western approach to sexuality. "From the fifth century on, Augustine's pessimistic views of sexuality, politics, and human nature would become the dominant influence of Western Christianity, both Catholic and Protestant, and color all Western culture, Christian or not, ever since" (p. 150). Or as D.P. Verene (1972) aptly puts it, many of Augustine's views on sexuality "seem surprisingly familiar to the attitudes we have absorbed since childhood simply by growing up in Western culture" (p. 86).

Augustine associated sexuality with the idea of original sin and the fall of humanity in the Garden of Eden. He proclaimed that sexual desire was the proof of—and penalty for—Adam's failure to resist temptation. Although men and women, according to the Christian tradition, are made in the image of God, their sexual urges show them to be a flawed and degenerate version of the deity. As Pagels (1988) suggests, "the Augustinian theory of original sin claims that our moral capacity has been so fatally infected that human nature as we know it cannot be trusted" (p. 149). From this perspective, sexuality is important for the survival of civilized society because it represents the moral weakness of humanity. Accordingly, it follows that as civilized societies attempt to control the "dark side" of human nature, they must place considerable emphasis on the regulation of sexuality. Western society has had a strong propensity to attempt to control sexual behaviour through both law and social norm. This tendency reflects the pervasive belief in the power and significance of sexuality in human affairs. "Every society, whether sexually permissive or restrictive, finds it useful and even necessary to regulate and structure its social relationships, especially sexual relations, in some way for the common good" (Shapiro & Francoeur, 1987, p. 88).

An important example of how Western society has structured social relationships by means of sexual regulation is the institution of the family. Since the Middle Ages, the nuclear family has been the dominant kinship grouping in Western society. The nuclear family is based, first and foremost, on the heterosexual union of a man and a woman bound together by a sexually monogamous relationship, providing Western society with a normative framework for producing children. The family unit has been designated as a central biological, social, political, and economic constituent of society. From their examination of the history of sexuality in the United States, D'Emilio and Freedman (1988) concluded that "In early America, a unitary system of sexual regulation that involved family, church, and state rested upon a consensus about the primacy of familial, reproductive sexuality" (p. xvii). While there can be no doubt that during the 20th century the links between sexuality, reproduction, and the family have loosened, they have not dissolved and many of the laws and social norms regulating sexuality in support of the nuclear family unit remain in force. One of the primary reasons they have persevered is because these sexual laws and norms preserve, for better or for worse, the existing social structure.

Many of the objections to an increasing trend toward the liberalization of sexual laws and norms are premised on the belief that a breakdown in traditional patterns of sexual regulation constitutes an assault on a way of life based on the sanctity of the nuclear family unit. The desire to regulate sexual behaviour in support of the family unit can be readily seen in the many laws that have been instituted in Western societies regarding such things as marriage, divorce, homosexuality, and prostitution, and in often strict social norms upholding practices such as premarital chastity, monogamy within marriage, and heterosexuality. Because family-oriented sexual ethics, based on Christian doctrine, have shaped the legal regulation of sexuality, it is not surprising that, for example, many American states continue to have laws proscribing sodomy between consenting adults, adultery, and fornication (Posner, 1992, pp. 77-78). As Gayle Rubin (cited in McCormick, 1994) notes "The only adult sexual behavior that is legal in every state of the union is the placement of the penis in the vagina in wedlock" (p. 7). For much of our history, including the present time, sexual laws and customs have supported the social ideal of the nuclear family.

Since the nuclear family has been basic to the organization of Western society, we can see how the regulation of sexuality plays a central role in maintaining the social order.

Social scientists from a diversity of disciplines have emphasized the importance of sexuality to Western society. While early Christian theologians connected sexuality with the sinful tendencies of humanity, 20th century psychology has attached a different but equally significant meaning to sexuality. One of this century's most influential figures, Sigmund Freud (1977), theorized about the centrality of sexuality in personality development and in so doing stressed "the importance of sexuality in all human achievements" (p. 43). Indeed, the psychological health of individuals and couples is now seen to be greatly dependant on sexual adjustment and fulfilment. James Nelson (1988) reflects this view of the importance of sexuality when he writes:

> Our sexuality is far more than genital activity. It is our way of being in the world as gendered persons, having male or female biological structures and socially internalized self-understandings of those meanings to us. Sexuality means having the capacity for sensuousness. Above all, sexuality is the desire for intimacy and communion, both emotionally and physically. It is the physiological and psychological grounding of our capacity to love. At its undistorted best, our sexuality is that basic eros of our humanness—urging, pulling, luring, driving us out of loneliness into communion, out of stagnation, into creativity. (p. 26)

This emphasis on the importance of sexual fulfilment and happiness has not detracted from the social or political significance of sexuality. In this view, sexual happiness is linked to the well-being of society. As George Frankl (1974) writes, "the root of human happiness is love, and sexual happiness is the foundation of social happiness, for he who cannot find sexual happiness cannot find love, and he who cannot find love cannot build a good society" (p. 13). The expansion of the meaning of sexuality beyond genital activity for the purposes of procreation is part of a shift in emphasis toward what sociologists call "affective individualism", the quest for personal fulfilment (Giddens, 1987). It has been argued that such a shift also has implications for the economic structure of society.

> The rise of "affective individualism" has been closely involved with the association of sexuality with personal fulfilment, inside and outside the

formal ties of marriage. Some radical writers have argued that the origins and continuation of capitalism are closely bound up psychologically with the repression of sexuality. The strict discipline demanded by industrial labour, in their view, is secured through the generalised curtailing of personal desires, epitomised by Victorian mores in the heyday of nineteenth-century capitalism. (Giddens, 1987, p. 130)

Herbert Marcuse (1966) is perhaps the most well-known theorist to propose a link between the social control of sexuality and the workings of capitalism, and other writers such as Wilhelm Reich (1962) have attempted to show that political liberation cannot occur without a complementary freedom from sexual repression. As Richard Posner (1992) suggests in an analysis of the legal regulation of sex in the United States,

We have seen that a number of sexual laws, and sexual customs having the force of law, including a variety of apparently senseless, seemingly vestigial sexual laws in this and other Anglo-Saxon societies (culturally although not ethnically, ours is still an Anglo-Saxon society), make sense—social-functional sense—when analyzed in economic terms. (p. 213)

One of the most provocative perspectives on the place of sexuality in the structuring of social life comes from philosopher Michel Foucault, who theorized that the organization of sexuality acts as a mechanism of power, operating as a means of control over bodies and identities. Foucault saw the history of sexuality as a history of discourses. By employing the term "discourses" Foucault was referring to organized bodies of knowledge which, when joined with the practice of theology, medicine, psychology, psychiatry, and the other human sciences, produce and transmit power. According to Foucault (1978), we have been engaged in a perpetual "will to knowledge" (p. 12), "speaking of it ad infinitum" (p. 35). The resulting discourses become mechanisms of power, ordering, classifying, and organizing the body's capacity for sensual pleasure into "polymorphous sexualities." Sexual identities, orientations, and perversions are formulated and come to define the individual and his/her behaviour. In sum, the discourses of knowledge-power become the reference points through which personal identities are constructed and social life is organized. For Foucault (1978), sexuality is "an especially dense transfer point for relations of power: between men and women, young people and old people, parents and offspring, teachers and students, priests and laity, an administration and a population" (p. 103). Sullivan (1995) succinctly states Foucault's position when he writes, "The history of sexuality in the West is not a history from repression to liberation, but the exchange of one kind of power relations for another" (p. 64).

Not only does the organization of sexuality continue to determine the nature of many of our key social institutions such as the family, but as Foucault suggested, sexuality has also increasingly come to define individual identity. This too has important ramifications for the nature of society. Biological sex and gender identity are arguably the most fundamental defining characteristics of the individual. The existence of the category of homosexuality "made the sexual significant by making it a signifying aspect of character" (Simon, 1994, p. 7). In the social world of our present culture, a person's sexual orientation is among the most salient features of how an individual is perceived by the self and others. It is at least as important as race, ethnicity and perhaps gender. More than any other event, the onset of puberty—the attainment of sexual and reproductive capacity—and subsequent experiences of sexual interaction, is seen as the clearest indication of the transition between childhood and adulthood. For many women, menopause, the cessation of reproductive capacity, is seen as a key marker in the shift from adulthood to old age.

Feminism, perhaps the most influential social movement of recent decades, also emphasizes the relationship between sexuality and the power to organize social life. This linkage between sexuality, gender equality, and social organization has, as Janice Irvine (1990) explains, been a central focus of the feminist movement.

> Although the feminism of the 1960s envisioned new strategies for organizing around sexual issues, this analysis reaffirmed that of feminists of the early 1900s: achieving sexual liberation for women was indistinguishable from changing wider sociopolitical power structures. (p. 137)

Feminism is grounded, in part, on the theory that the inequality of women is expressed through the gender specific codes of sexual behaviour inherent in the patriarchal social system (e.g., Brownmiller, 1975; Steedman, 1987; Vance, 1984). Feminists such as Catherine Mackinnon (1982) identify sexuality as "the primary social sphere of male power" (p. 529). In sum, "Sexuality is important, feminists argue, because *norms* regarding 'proper' and 'normal' sexual behavior function everywhere to socialize and control women's behavior" (Tiefer, 1995, p. 114).

This brief survey of different perspectives toward the importance attached to sexuality leads to two basic conclusions. First, from early Judeo-Christian theological scholars to contemporary feminists, virtually every social scientist who has seriously examined the cultural implications of human sexuality, in one or all of its multiplicity of dimensions, arrives at the conclusion that, in one way or another, the sexual norms of a particular culture provide a central pivot upon which much of the social, political, and even economic character of that culture is derived. In other words, sexuality is important in that its organization significantly shapes the nature of society. In Eve Sedgwick's words (cited in Stanton, 1992), sexuality is "the most meaning intensive of human activities" (p. 2), or as Stephan Jay Gould (cited in Stanton, 1992) puts it, sexuality is "a sign, a symbol, or reflection of nearly everything in our culture" (p. 2).

Second, the history of sexuality is a history of change. For example, as we have seen, whereas Augustine saw sexuality as the expression of human weakness and immorality, contemporary psychology sees sexuality as vital to human happiness. The enormity of this difference in perspective is summed up well by Thomas Szasz (1980) when he suggests that "To the great doctor of Christianity in the fourth century, sexual desire was a disease; to the great doctors of coitus today, lack of sexual desire is a disease" (p. xi). Put another way, "...the dominant meaning of sexuality has changed during our history from a primary association with reproduction within families to a primary association with emotional intimacy and physical pleasure for individuals" (D'Emilio & Freedman, 1988, p. xv).

As a result, increasingly large segments of Western society have come to accept the legitimacy of sexual acts that occur outside the context of reproduction within marriage. Simply put, the meaning attached to sexuality has been undergoing a profound transformation characterized by the emergence of a mixture of diverse sexual norms and values that has replaced the uniformity of the past. Although it is more than likely that the sexual uniformity that we commonly associate with pre-1960s Western culture is somewhat overstated, there can be no doubt that the growing acceptance of sexuality beyond its traditional familial reproductive function has lead to an ever increasing variability in the meaning and perceived role of sexuality in our lives. Today, more than ever, sex means different things to different people, and the moral, social, and psychological ramifications of engaging in any given sexual act can be very different depending on who you are and what you believe.

However, these transformations in the meaning of sexuality have been neither smooth nor complete. Indeed, the existence of these divergent meaning systems related to sexuality has been a major focus of what is often referred to as the "culture wars." Because sexuality and the societal norms related to it carry such significance for the shape of society itself, sexuality has become the site of considerable social and moral conflict. While large segments of Western society remain strongly attached to what might be described as a traditional view of sexuality based on reproduction within the family unit, a significant proportion of society believes that a dismantling of traditional sexual values, replacing them with a set of values that emphasize sexual and reproductive freedom, will lead to a more just society. The schism in the views of sexual morality in contemporary America has been made abundantly clear in surveys on what sexual activities people believe are morally acceptable. For example, according to a recent, nationally representative survey, 19.7% of Americans believe that premarital sex is always wrong. In addition, 60.8% believe that teenage participation in premarital sex is always wrong and 64.8% believe that homosexual sex is always wrong (Laumann, Gagnon, Michael, & Michaels, 1994, p. 514; Michael, Gagnon, Laumann, & Kolata, 1994, p. 234). In other words, while about 60% of people resolutely reject the moral acceptability of homosexuality and premarital sex among teenagers, close to 40% do not, indicating that large segments of society disagree with each other on this issue. The authors of this survey concluded from their findings that "aspects or consequences of sexual behavior such as sex before marriage, abortion, and homosexuality are among the social issues about which we as a nation seem to have no clear consensus at this time" (Laumann, et al., 1994, p. 547). A Kinsey Institute survey of Americans' beliefs about sexual morality, conducted in the 1970s, provides further evidence of clear divisions on these issues. In the Kinsey Institute survey, while 56.4% of respondents believed that "premarital sex by a teenage boy with a girl he loves" is always or almost always wrong, 42.8% felt that it was wrong only sometimes or not wrong at all. While 70% disapproved of homosexual activity even when the participants were in love, close to 30% believed there were circumstances when homosexual sex had the potential for moral acceptability (Klassen, Williams & Levitt, 1989, p. 18). In addition, 59.1% believed that homosexuality should be against the law while 37.8% stated their opposition to the legal proscription of homosexual acts (Klassen, Williams & Levitt, 1989, p. 173). What is apparent from these findings is that while a little over half of Americans seem to believe that certain sexual acts are intrinsically or always wrong, a sizable proportion of Americans look to the context or circumstances in which a sexual act takes place before proceeding to make a moral judgement about it.

Although there have been no systematic, large scale national studies on the sexual attitudes and beliefs of Canadians, available data support the conclusion that while many Canadians continue to hold conservative views of sexual conduct, "more Canadians in the 1990's than in prior years accept, or are at least tolerant of, a wider diversity of forms of sexual conduct, expression and communication" (Barrett, King, Levy, Maticka-Tyndale, & McKay, 1997, p. 236).

Overall, these numbers indicate a clear lack of consensus within the North American public on issues of sexual morality. In addition, they also suggest that although Western society has passed through numerous scientific, political, philosophical, and demographic transformations, including at least one "sexual revolution" since the ascension of the Augustinian view of sexuality, many, if not most, Americans continue to adhere to the traditional Christian moral perspective on sexuality. This perseverance of traditional views of sexual morality exists simultaneously with a growing trend of revolt against traditional values on the part of many groups, including feminists, gay and lesbian rights activists, and those who might generally be described as embracing secular humanist values and/or liberal theological interpretations of sexual morality. Although most Americans apparently continue to adhere to a traditional sexual morality, since the 1960s, in particular, "Many more Americans than before liberalized their views on masturbation, premarital relations, extramarital affairs, homosexuality, and began to forgive themselves and others for engaging in previously tabooed acts" (Ellis, 1990, p. 6).

These divergent meaning systems do not peacefully co-exist in an open market place of ideas and lifestyles. The mere existence of one meaning system in the public sphere is perceived as a threat to the way of life based on another meaning system. The clash between the traditional Christian and contemporary secular moral perspectives on sexuality as they pertain to sex and gender roles and homosexuality illustrates why these seemingly mutually exclusive meaning systems have been unable to peacefully co-exist. From the traditional Christian point of view both feminism and the homosexual rights movements seek to destroy the family as we know it. According to the feminist and homosexual rights movements, the traditional Western organization of social life is oppressive for women and gays and lesbians.

The degree to which feminist perspectives on sexuality have been the subject of intense social science and media discussion and debate is an example of the power of sexuality related issues to provoke disagreements. While nearly everyone would agree that the implications of sexual changes related to sex and gender are immense, the direction that society ought to take in the organization of sex and gender is hotly contested. For example, the changing nature of sex roles, partially embodied by male and female scripts for sexual behaviour, are seen as an important issue because, as Robert Francoeur (1987) suggests, "Sex roles and conformity to those roles are essential if an individual is to relate to and be accepted as a part of the whole society. Sex roles allow us to maintain a stable society" (p. 29). In addition, sex role arrangements, even in societies that are stable, need to be viewed in terms of their ability to protect individual rights, ensure equality between groups, and to benefit society as a whole. Those with a traditional view believe that

> The differences between the sexes are the single most important fact of human society. The drive to deny them—in the name of women's liberation, marital openness, sexual equality, erotic consumption, homosexual romanticism—must be one of the most quixotic crusades in the history of the species. Yet in a way it is typical of crusades. For it is a crusade against a particular incarnate humanity—men and women and children—on behalf of a metaphysical "humanism." (Gilder, 1987, p. 37)

According to this perspective, allowing women to explore avenues of sexual freedom which for many may lie outside the confines of marriage, and to have easy access to contraceptives and abortion, tempts women away from participation in the nuclear family structure, a trend which is seen to be detrimental to society.

According to many feminists, the patriarchal family and the sexual norms that support it are at the root of gender oppression. Feminists, therefore, have encouraged women to explore alternatives to traditional family life and the roles that men and women play within it. Many feminist social scientists believe that gender differences, and their complementary sex roles, do not reflect incarnate humanity but are "best explained as a social construction rooted in hierarchy" (Fuchs Epstien, 1988, p. 15), created by patriarchal society in order to institutionalize male privilege. As noted above, many feminists contend that this gender hierarchy is embedded in the sexual world, requiring a dismantling of traditional sexual scripts that emphasize male assertiveness and female passivity and a double standard toward sexual freedom. Reshaping the sexual aspects of gender arrangements is a key aspect of feminism's goal to create a gender equal society. These two competing conceptions of sex roles are seen to be mutually exclusive in that one can only gain in influence at the expense of the other.

Those who follow the traditional Christian view of sexuality have been unable to affirm the moral validity of homosexuality because they see it as not only against the laws of God and nature but also because they see homosexuality as a dangerous threat to a way of life based on the family. Naturally, those who favour equal rights for homosexuals are unable to accept this version of Christian doctrine because they see it as discriminatory against gay and lesbian people. In effect the feminist and homosexual rights movements have undermined

> the "naturalness" and inevitability of traditional gender stereotypes and the monolithic nuclear family. And whereas feminism had affirmed nonreproductive sexuality, gay sexuality involved an explicit separation of sex and reproduction, which foregrounded the option of sex solely for pleasure. By their very existence, gay people challenge the "principle of consistency," which links sex, gender, and sexual preference in a socially normative ideal. (Irvine, 1990, p. 139)

As Schur (1988) notes we can see here the logic behind the belief held by many traditionalists that "If homosexuality is 'allowed,' that will be the end of the family as we know it" (p. 19). It reflects an assumption that if membership in the nuclear family, and acceptance of the moral codes governing the sexuality of the family unit, become optional rather than compulsory, the nuclear family will disappear as a social institution.

Homosexuality and sex/gender roles are but two of a number of sexually related issues that are a source of intense social conflict. The pressures for, and resistance to, sexual change can be seen in the deep divisions within Western society on issues such as premarital sex, pornography, contraception, strategies for AIDS prevention, prostitution, and sexuality education in the schools. Because sexuality is considered so important, changes in sexual norms and values are often resisted by large segments of society. This is not surprising since as sexual norms and values change, society itself is changed in fundamental ways. Since sexuality is not a simple or unified phenomenon, but rather an extraordinarily complex and varied one with a multitude of profound implications for the ordering of social life, sexuality has become a major battleground in a cultural war between competing value systems. As D'Emilio and Freedman (1988) note, by the 1980s, this clash of value systems had reached a new high point of intensity.

> The debates about sex, rather than remaining the province of feminist and gay liberationists, were polarizing the nation's politics. The contentious quality of the debates stemmed not only from the demands of radicals, but also from conservatives distressed by the reorientation of sexual values that had occurred since the 1960s. The sexual politics of the New Right, as well as more recent controversies generated by the AIDS epidemic, attest to how deeply sexuality had infiltrated national politics by the 1980s. (p. 345)

By the mid 1990s, Western culture's continued inability to cope with and agree upon solutions to a growing plethora of sexually related social problems, including epidemics of AIDS and other sexually transmitted diseases, gender conflict and inequality, sexual violence and abuse, oppression of sexual minorities, and high rates of unwanted adolescent pregnancy, reflect and exacerbate increasingly volatile social conflict surrounding sexuality. As Weeks (1986) puts it,

> There is a struggle for the future of sexuality. But the ways we respond to this have been coloured by the force of the accumulated historical heritage and sexual traditions out of which we have come: The Christian organization of belief in sex as subversive, the liberal belief in sex as source of identity and personal resource, all rooted in a melange of religious, scientific and sexological arguments about what sex is, what it can do, and what we must and must not do. (p. 5)

The very nature of society is believed to be at stake in this battle between competing views of the nature, function, and moral aspects of human sexuality.

Sexuality Education

There are many factors which can contribute to socio-sexual changes in our society. According to Gagnon and Simon (1973), "Changes in the sexual component of the human condition can result from changes in the biological, technological, and psychosocial domains of life" (p. 287). Shifts in the demographic structure of society (i.e., expanding urbanization, ethno-cultural mixing, changing age ratios, etc.), rapid advances in communication technologies resulting in easier access to sexual information, growth in our scientific understanding of human sexuality, technological advances related to sexuality such as better and more effective birth control and countless other factors can affect the way we think and behave sexually. The advent of birth control, in particular, has been cited as a major agent of social change. As Money and Tucker (1975) argue, "The ability to separate the bait of sexual pleasure from the hook of reproduction sparked a revolution more momentous for the human race than any in history" (p. 186). Although, as we have seen, many people continue to share the sexual views of Augustine, Hatfield and Rapson (1993) note that by the late 18th century, changes in the material, economic, political, philosophical, and psychological spheres of Western society had begun to fundamentally alter the fabric of the Western world and many of these changes have unavoidably resulted in "a metamorphosis in Euro-American approaches to love and sex" (p. 87). In sum, many shifts in sexual beliefs, customs, laws, and behaviours can be viewed as more or less rational adaptations to changing socio-historical contingencies.

However, given that sexuality has been imbued with monumental social significance, it is not surprising that conscious attempts to socialize youth in sexual matters have become such a decisive and controversial issue. If we define socialization as the process by which social authorities and institutions transmit to children the beliefs, values, and behaviours deemed appropriate to a particular culture, a bitter debate about the sexual socialization of youth is a highly significant and natural outgrowth of the sexual conflicts that now permeate Western culture.

In order to harmoniously participate in society, an individual must internalize and adhere to the ground rules of the social reality of that society. "The ontogenetic process by which this is brought about is socialization, which may thus be defined as the comprehensive and consistent induction of an individual into the objective world of a society or sector of it" (Berger

& Luckmann, 1967, p. 130). And, as Berger and Luckmann (1967) note, even human activities which are "grounded in biological drives," such as sexual behaviour, are subject, through the socialization process, to "the social channelling of activity" (p. 181). Indeed, it has been argued that "nothing is more essentially transmitted by a social process of learning than sexual behavior" (Douglas cited in Stanton, 1992, p. 4). In their analysis of adolescent sexuality, Zabin and Hayward (1993) note that "Young men and women adopt sexual behaviors at a time that is influenced by hormonal development, but they follow a script that is largely determined by social expectations" (p. 41).

Thus, there is reason to believe that, while historical forces inevitably influence sexual norms, conscious effort to shape the sexual socialization of youth, either in accordance with or against historical trends, will significantly affect the beliefs and behaviour of emerging generations. But as cultural diversity in sexual norms and values becomes more and more of a reality in Western culture, a clearly articulated and widely agreed upon set of reference points from which the sexual socialization of youth can proceed becomes exceedingly difficult to identify.

The sources of sexual socialization are numerous. For example, research has shown that a number of "important variables affect sexual knowledge, attitudes, and behavior including peer attitudes and behavior, family of origin values, self-efficacy, locus of control, choice of partner, relationship with partner, and media exposure" (Dine Jacobs & Wolf, 1995, p. 91). However, it is with sexuality education in the schools that our society makes its most concerted attempt to employ a public institution to socialize youth in regard to the sexual norms and mores of our culture. There is considerable evidence that some school-based sexuality education programs have influenced students' sexual knowledge, attitudes, and some aspects of their behaviour (Kirby, 1993; Kirby, et al., 1994; Mellanby, Phelps, Crichton, & Tripp, 1995; Frost & Forrest, 1995; Mauldon & Luker, 1996). Thus, it is not surprising that with the diverse plurality of moral perspectives on the meaning of sexuality, the picture of human sexuality to be presented in the public school classroom is fertile ground for what has become a polarized debate. After all, "Visions of what is considered 'good education' are intimately rooted in the conscious and/or unconscious visions of what is considered a 'good society'" (Goodman, 1992, p. xix).

Thomas Szasz (1980) shows how sexuality education has come to be seen as a battle between seemingly irreconcilable moral perspectives on the sexual socialization of youth when he writes:

> Since human behavior denotes the actions of moral agents, all behavior is, in part at least, a matter of ethics. Sexual behavior is very much a matter of ethics. Hence, since time immemorial, persons who proposed to teach people about sex had but two choices: to embrace and endorse the accepted, traditional sexual ways of the group, or to explore and enjoin sexual principles and practices at odds with those ways. There is no such thing as value free sex education, nor can there be. (pp. 99-100)

Sharon Thompson (1994) writes that "Sex education is potentially a vehicle for social engineering par excellence, be it progressive or traditional" (p. 40). As Philip Meredith (1989) suggests, in one view, sexuality education should "recommend self-control over the force within in order to ensure the survival of the marriage bond, the family, and by extension society itself, from collapse" (p. 45). Yet from another perspective, sexuality education may be able to impart "the capacity and courage to look critically at social arrangements, to chart out rigorous spaces analysis of power, to seek out intellectual and political surprises" (Philips and Fine, 1992, p. 249). Given its potential role in shaping the sexual-moral landscape, it is not surprising that sexuality education has become arguably the most crucial battle in the cultural war over sexuality.

Until relatively recently, the validity of providing sexuality education in the schools was suspect for a number of reasons. Primary among them was the widely held assumption that it was inappropriate to discuss sexuality with children. Such discussion, it was believed, would corrupt youthful innocence and predispose children to immoral behaviour. In addition, teaching about sexuality in an open forum such as the public school classroom violated a cultural taboo on any form of public discussion of sexuality. Most importantly, since the formal sexuality education of youth, when it existed in any direct or tangible sense, was considered to be the exclusive domain of the family and church, school-based sexuality education has, as we have seen, raised difficult and controversial questions about which set of norms and values will be taught in the classroom.

In most respects, all but the last of these concerns has dissipated with the growing recognition in principle that we must equip young people with the means to understand and protect their own reproductive health and potential: and that rapid changes taking place in society demand that parents and churches be assisted in this through the formal educational process. (Meredith, 1989, p. 1)

The question of whether sexuality should be hidden from youth is now more or less moot as various forms of media continually expose youth to sexually-oriented imagery. Thus, many of those formerly opposed to school-based sexuality education now contend that it is necessary in order to counter what are seen as the overly permissive messages and mores propagated by the popular media.

Since the advent of the AIDS crisis, the need for sexuality education in the schools has become almost universally accepted. Surveys in both the United States (Gallup Poll, 1985, 1991; Janus & Janus, 1993; Louis Harris Associates, 1988; Welshimer & Harris, 1994) and Canada (Lawlor & Purcell, 1988; Marsmen & Herold, 1986; McKay, 1996; Ornstein, 1989; Verby & Herold, 1992) indicate that the vast majority of adults, including parents of school age children, approve of sexuality and/or AIDS education in the schools. For example, a 1991 survey of a national sample of American adults indicated that 87% approved of sexuality education in the schools (Gallup, 1991). In a national sample of American adults, Janus and Janus (1993) found that only 1% of respondents were adamantly opposed to sexuality education in the schools while 90% were "definitely" in favour (p. 97). Perhaps most notable was the finding that 89% of those respondents who were categorized as "ultraconservative" were "definitely" in favour of sexuality education in the schools (p. 280).

Access to sexuality education, particularly as it relates to the prevention of disease and exploitation, is increasingly seen as a necessary and basic right of the individual. The World Health Organization (WHO) proclaims that "sexuality influences thoughts, feelings, actions, and interactions and thereby our mental and physical health. Since health is a fundamental human right, so must sexual health also be a basic human right" (WHO, cited in Health Canada, 1994, p. 7). If sexual health, as a key component of overall health, can legitimately be considered a fundamental human right, it may also be reasonably argued that the denial of the opportunity to learn the information and skills necessary to protect and enhance one's sexual health is tantamount to a violation of this human right.

However, as Meredith (1989) suggests, "The problems which follow from a 'formalisation' of what has traditionally been a hidden, furtive, taboo-ridden, even unconscious area of learning for many are many and complex" (p. 1). So, as Bruess and Greenberg (1994) note, "in recent years the sexuality education controversy has centred more on the content and methodology of programs rather than on whether or not there should be a program" (p. 57). Much of this controversy centres around different perspectives on the value positions reflected in contemporary sexuality education, and on what those positions should be. For example, Barrett (1994) summarizes this tension in Canadian sexuality education as follows:

> Canadians appear to be strongly supportive of the schools involvement in sexuality education. Nevertheless, a sizable minority views contemporary sex education as skewed toward liberal, secular attitudes, particularly in the areas of abortion, homosexuality, teen sexuality, and access to contraceptive information and services, and actively promulgates a more restrictive agenda in all of these areas. Although historically this view has been expressed as an opposition to sexuality education in the schools, at present it is more likely to focus on either the specific value positions that schools should adopt, the appropriateness of particular topics (e.g. homosexuality, contraception, abortion), or the ways in which student behaviour should be influenced (e.g. abstinence-only programs). (pp. 200-201)

There have been many different objectives proposed for sexuality education in the schools. Among the more common, and sometimes contested, objectives are instilling a basic knowledge of human reproductive physiology, clarifying values, increasing social skills, learning methods of expressing affection, increasing comfort with communication about sexuality, enhancing self-esteem, and reducing exploitation (Kirby, 1992). It has also been proposed in some quarters that sexuality education should encourage a critique of prevailing gender roles as they pertain to sexuality so that students may have a greater opportunity to build more egalitarian relationships than those prescribed by patriarchy (e.g., Fine, 1988; Szirom, 1988). A small number of sex educators have increasingly focussed on reducing homophobia and have begun to recognize the sex education needs of gay and lesbian students (e.g., Sears, 1992). These latter two objectives have been, as we might expect, highly controversial. In any case,

> ...educators in the field of sexuality inevitably do their work under some assumptions about its purpose and value—assumptions that

include a particular vision of the place of sexuality in social behavior
in general and the needs of teenagers in particular. (Zabin & Hayward,
1993, p. 113)

Despite the controversy over the objectives of sexuality education in
the schools, nearly all programs do intend, in some way, to provide information that will help students reduce or eliminate their risk of unintended
pregnancy, or STD infection with a particular emphasis being placed on
HIV/AIDS. Indeed, any account of contemporary sexuality education in
the schools cannot be divorced from the fact that a major priority is to help
young people avoid sexual problems such as unintended pregnancy and
infection with sexually transmitted diseases. The emergence of HIV/AIDS
has added an unprecedented urgency to what can be described as sexuality
education's public health mandate. With a focus on the pragmatic aspects
of pregnancy and disease prevention, one might expect that the public
controversy around sexuality education in the schools would be diminished.

However, proposals for how problems, such as pregnancy and STD
prevention among youth, should be addressed both pedagogically in the
classroom and in the larger society are closely interwoven with one's views
on sexual morality. So, for example, if I have qualms about the moral
acceptability of premarital sex, I might favour sexual education for adolescents that emphasizes sexual abstinence outside of marriage. If I think that
sex outside of marriage can be morally acceptable, I may be more likely to
sympathize with educational programs that encourage sexually active youth
to use contraception and practise safer sex. In sum, whether one bemoans
the lack of emphasis on a "Just Say No" to sex approach in contemporary
sexuality education or complains that sexuality education fails to sufficiently
acknowledge the positive aspects of safer sex practices will largely depend
on where one lines up in the cultural battle over the future of sexuality in
our society. In other words, if it is true that sexuality education cannot be
value free, it would also appear that even seeking to achieve commonly
shared objectives like preventing unwanted pregnancy and sexually transmitted diseases is a morally laden and divisive enterprise.

Conclusion

When communities battle over sexuality education in the schools, it is
not simply a minor quibble over the effectiveness of particular educational
methodologies. Although the question of what works in terms of pregnancy

and STD prevention is a hotly debated topic (McKay, 1992), when battles over sexuality education occur, they reflect a clash of fundamental values, of different ways of seeing the world. In short, it is a struggle between ideologies in general and a clash of sexual ideologies in particular. The essence and true character of the sexuality education question becomes more visible when it is understood in the context of ideology.

CHAPTER TWO

Restrictive and Permissive Sexual Ideologies

― ‥ ― ‥ ― ‥ ― ‥ ― ‥ ―‥ ‥ı

> "People are deeply divided about human nature—including the nature of human sexuality."
>
> (Mosher, 1989)

> "Ideology typically fixes meaning, naturalizing or externalizing its prevailing forms by putting them beyond question, and thereby also effacing the contradictions and conflicts of the social domain."
>
> (Dollimore, 1991)

> "The forces of liberation or chaos, depending on your vantage point, stand against the forces of repression or civilized morality. Sexuality has become a battlefield where opponents rally their troops against a demonized enemy."
>
> (Seidman, 1992)

Introduction

Jorge Larrain (1979) describes ideology as "one of the most equivocal and elusive concepts one can find in social sciences" (p. 1). The social science literature contains a multitude of meanings given to ideology. Thompson (1984) in *Studies in the Theory of Ideology* simplifies things considerably by delineating two fundamentally different ways the concept of ideology is defined in the social science literature. On one hand, "ideology is essentially linked to the process of sustaining asymmetrical relations of power—that is, to the process of maintaining domination" (Thompson, 1984, p. 4). In this sense, ideology carries a negative connotation, linking ideology to the process of critique. Hence Thompson calls this perspective the *critical conception* of ideology.

There is another conception of ideology which is perhaps more commonplace, and descriptive in its meaning. In this other view, ideologies are seen as systems of thought and belief and/or of symbolic practices that inform social action or political projects. According to Thompson (1984),

> No attempt is made on the basis of this conception, to distinguish between the kinds of action or projects which ideology animates; ideology is present in every political programme, irrespective of whether the program is directed towards the preservation or transfor-mation of the social order. (p. 4)

This approach is what Thompson calls a *neutral conception* of ideology.

I will adopt a *neutral conception* of ideology to analyze the relation between sexual ideology and sexuality education in the schools. While the beliefs inherent within a particular sexual ideology may contribute to asymmetrical relations of power, I intend to look at sexual ideologies as unified systems of belief, focussing on their normative character rather than on their empirical or moral validity. I will treat ideologies, to use Mosher's (1991) words, as "...systems of belief about the nature of the world and of humankind that define and frame 'reality'" (p. 7).

Ideologies have a variety of functions. They provide us with a cognitive structure around which we can organize our thoughts into a unified, logically consistent set of beliefs about the world and of humanity. A primary function of ideology is to provide a framework that gives our beliefs order, coherence, and consistency. As Greenberg (1988) puts it,

> As people live in society, they grapple with and try to come to terms with it. In so doing, they develop ideologies that explain, justify, or challenge it. Possibly they act on the basis of their ideologies. Their actions generate exposure to new experiences, which may induce them to modify their previously held beliefs. Of course, the ideas so devel-oped need not be a direct unmediated reflection of a social reality. In general, people interpret experience in light of previous ideas and conceptual schemes, not with a mental tabula rasa. (p. 18)

Ideologies may be held dispassionately and unreflectively as a set of taken-for-granted assumptions about the nature of things or, in the case of what Hoffer (1951) calls the true believer, an ideology may be held with a passionate fervour.

Ideologies have other important functions. An ideology, as a system of belief, unites the individuals who share it, giving them a sense of solidarity and collective purpose. It is in this way that the members of social-political movements achieve their identity as part of a wider community of people with similar beliefs. An ideology can tell us who we are, and just as importantly, who we are not. Mosher (1991) writes that

> Ideology binds us together and divides us from the Other as a nation, as a religion, and as a gender. We become one, a union, a unity of shared believers, invidiously contrasted to the Other who holds those foreign and false beliefs, who can't see the forest for the trees, can't see the end of their own noses, can't see the way things truly are. (pp. 7-8)

A third but equally important function of ideology is to cement the ideologue's convictions in the face of uncertainty. As a system of beliefs, an ideology can provide us with an epistemological framework for addressing philosophical questions that are not amenable to empirical verification. Questions about the existence of God or which is the best political creed are examples of philosophical questions to which there are no objectively certain answers. An ideology entails a unified set of intellectual, social, and moral constructs that manifest themselves in a belief system with an internalized logical consistency, providing a secure foundation for how we approach such questions. When these constructs are strong and consistent enough they can imbue an ideology with the power to define reality for those who are true believers. In his analysis of the true believer in mass movements, Hoffer (1951) illustrates the dynamics through which an ideology provides certainty of belief.

> All active mass movements strive, therefore, to interpose a fact-proof screen between the faithful and the realities of the world. They do this by claiming that the ultimate and absolute truth is already embodied in their doctrine and that there is no truth nor certitude outside it. The facts on which the true believer bases his conclusions must not be derived from his experience or observation but from holy writ. (p. 78)

In other words, "Whatever his sanctified line, the true believer is wholly convinced he or she is acting in the very best interests of both the proximate and ultimate truth" (Hentoff, 1992, p. 57). Within the ideologically constructed reality, explanations that are congruent with the ideology's logic seem plausible and eminently reasonable. Thus, the theory of creationism seems reasonable to many devout Christians and the theory of evolution seems reasonable to the secular Humanist. In other words, ideology defines reality, not vice versa.

Ideologies encompass a wide spectrum of beliefs: religious, political, social, etc. Beliefs about sexuality fall into the ideological realm. As a subset of ideology, sexual ideology "refers to an individual's beliefs and attitudes regarding the regulation and expression of sexual conduct" (Troiden & Platt-Jendrek, 1987, p. 257). Questions about the nature of human sexuality, its purpose, its proper role in human relationships, and the moral guidelines that ought to govern its conduct are invariably addressed in an ideological context. One's ideas about the moral validity of homosexual relationships, for example, are based on subjective conviction rather than objectively observable facts. One's views about homosexuality can take on the veneer of objectivity when immersed within an ideological belief system. Hence, within the ideological reality of the fundamentalist Christian, homosexuality is sometimes seen to be, in an objective sense, unnatural, contrary to the word of God, and therefore immoral. To those of a contrary ideological persuasion, that line of reasoning has nothing to do with objective reality. Indeed, using biological sex as a criterion for the moral evaluation of a sexual relationship would be seen, in this alternate view, as patently absurd. Other criteria such as the potential for mutual fulfilment and respect would be considered far more important in judging the moral validity of a sexual relationship than the sex of the participants. When ideological perspectives, such as these, collide, the resulting disputes

> almost invariably deteriorate into bitter rhetorical and social battles. Sexual differences seem to automatically escalate into sex wars.... These skirmishes on the sexual front escalate as sexual and intimate affairs get entangled with nonsexual interests and conflicts. As sexual issues like pornography, homosexuality, S/M and casual sex are interpreted as signs or symptoms of the social state of America, sexual conflicts assume a heightened moral and political interest. (Seidman, 1992, pp. 7-8)

Because ideologies are social constructions with highly variable conceptions of reality, a contest between sexual ideologies—a testing of their respective validity—is a fight between combatants who are often competing on different conceptual playing fields. They are, in effect, attempting to play the same game but with different rules. This is so because "the world views that underlie sexual interpretations are not held rationally, but rather are the very conditions of rationality" (Davis, 1983, p. 230). When we present arguments to a person that are outside his or her ideological belief system, we are unlikely to change his or her mind. It is tantamount to asking them to transform their perception of reality. Thus, it is unlikely, for example, that Jerry Falwell, Pat Robertson, and their millions of followers will one day renounce their belief that homosexuality is morally wrong and gay and lesbian rights activists are not likely to give up their belief that homosexual relationships are in every way just as legitimate as heterosexual unions.

Perhaps because its popular culture is suffused with sexual imagery, Western society seems to be permeated by ideological conflict around issues of sexuality: homosexuality, premarital and extramarital sex, teenage sexuality, contraception, and pornography, to name a few. A number of typologies may be used to classify the players in these ideological disputes. While some sexual ideologies clearly represent different ends of a continuum of ideologies (hedonist and religious fundamentalist views about sexuality for example), many ideological beliefs about sexuality are only distinguishable by subtle shades of difference. A meticulous representation of these belief systems would therefore require the identification of a multiplicity of discreet sexual ideologies. This is so because "Sexual attitudes are strongly influenced by subcultural norms in general and religion in particular, by sociopolitical ideology, SES, and to a lesser extent, gender, and family structure" (Smith, 1994, p. 94). To the extent that different belief systems are mediated by individual characteristics such as personal history, gender, age, race, religion, socioeconomic status, and sexual orientation, the possible permutations of sexual ideology become infinite. For the purposes of clarity, most scholarship describing the conflict between sexual ideologies has emphasized ideological polarities or divided the ideological groupings into two or three broad categories. For example, Davis (1983) contrasts the Jehovanist with the Naturalist sexual ideology, Weeks (1985, 1986) looks at the Absolutist, Liberal and Libertarian, and Seidman (1992) dichotomizes the Romanticist and Libertarian ideologies.

In the remainder of this chapter, I use a synthesis of these typologies to provide a categorical framework for analyzing ideological perspectives on sexuality education. This synthesis yields two opposing perspectives which I term the Restrictive and Permissive sexual ideologies. In my view, the Jehovanist, Absolutist, and Romanticist ideologies described by these authors share a restrictive approach to human sexuality, whereas the Naturalist, Liberal and Libertarian ideologies are united by an emphasis on the assumed virtue of varying degrees of sexual freedom which, when compared to restrictive approaches, can be described as permissive. The views of religious traditionalists from various faiths, social-political conservatives, and radical feminists are generally encompassed by Restrictive sexual ideology. They advocate sexual ethics that prescribe strict limitations on sexual behaviour when compared to Permissive sexual ideology. In contrast, secular humanists, social-political liberals, and liberal feminists are representative of Permissive sexual ideology in that their views are generally less directive in terms of sexual ethics and behaviour.

At a superficial level, the division between Restrictive and Permissive sexual ideology can be understood in terms of the more familiar differentiation between the conservative and the liberal in that, "Conservatives tend to value order, individual responsibility, and control, while liberals are more likely to value variety and personal freedom" (Eisenman, 1994, p. 75). (Radical feminism may constitute an exception to this form of categorization, depending on whether one considers Radical feminists to be more liberal or more conservative.) Although conservatives typically discourage government intervention in the economic environment, there is as Eisenman (1994) notes,

> one area where conservatives tend to want government interference, in order to produce more order and control. That is the area of sexual behavior. Many conservatives see sexual freedom as an evil that can lead to the decline of the society. (p. 75)

Research on the correlates of individual attitudes towards sexuality suggests that those with a liberal political philosophy have a greater acceptance of sexual permissiveness (Smith, 1994). "This may indicate that those adopting a general liberal philosophy apply broad principles such as tolerance and individual choice to the sexual arena and that support for sexual freedom is seen as a liberal tenet" (Smith, 1994, p. 83).

Although I will present detailed accounts of the various permutations of the Restrictive and Permissive sexual ideologies, I am fully aware that these classifications are imperfect. Since our beliefs about sexuality often have complex and sometimes contradictory origins, no typology or classification system can avoid representing ideal types rather than the specific, multifaceted belief systems of unique individuals. Nevertheless, my classification of sexual beliefs into Restrictive and Permissive sexual ideologies does, to borrow a phrase from Andrew Sullivan (1995) "delineate the essential contours of the debate" (p. 20) over how our society should approach sexuality in general and sexuality education in particular. They do, as I hope to show, hold enough currency as general categories to help us make sense out of the debate and to move forward in resolving it.

Restrictive Sexual Ideology

The origins of Restrictive sexual ideology can easily be traced to early Christianity and its biblically oriented negative perception of human sexuality. Augustine set the tone for Western perspectives on sexuality through his interpretation of Adam and Eve's action in the Garden of Eden, and it is at this point that Murray Davis (1983) locates the beginnings of what he calls Jehovanist sexual ideology.

> Adam and Eve were the first to sift their sexual experience through Jehovanism's conceptual and moral mesh. In other words, they suddenly realized that their world was divided into two realms—a "good" everyday realm and an "evil" erotic realm—and that they had to suppress the latter as much as possible by concealing the physical features that generated it. (p. 166)

In this view, Adam and Eve's donning of fig leaves to cover their genitals symbolized the shamefulness of their sexuality. Sexual desire was condemned for its propensity to drag the self downward toward the earthly realm, preventing it from flowing upward towards God. Davis (1983) labels this perspective toward sexuality *Jehovanist* "after the name for the God of the Old Testament who becomes especially wrathful whenever his lawful category system is violated by sex or other tabooed activity" (p. 95). This Jehovanist view of sexuality reflected "a more general asceticism which accused all physical pleasure of diverting attention away from the highly valued spiritual realm toward the lowly valued material realm" (Davis, 1983, p. 167). As Christianity became the dominant Western world view, the condemnation of sexuality became all pervasive. Davis (1983) cites Kant as an example of how Western philosophical discourse adopted an anti-sexual perspective. "Kant saw sex as undermining the essential distinction between human beings and beasts" (Davis, 1983, p. 170). In his *Lectures on Ethics*, Kant (cited in Davis, 1983) proclaimed that

> All men and women do their best to make more alluring not their humanity but their sex, and direct their activities and lust entirely toward the latter. Humanity is thereby sacrificed to sex....By making human nature an instrument to satisfy their lusts, they dishonor it by

lowering it to the level of animal nature. Sexuality, therefore, exposes
mankind to the danger of equality with beast. (p. 170)

With this statement, Kant expressed the core premise of Jehovanist sexual
ideology: sexuality is a negative force, polluting and corrupting human
nature, and should therefore be reserved solely for procreation. Once this
core principle of Jehovanist sexual ideology was established, the ethics
governing human sexual conduct followed logically. Because of its propensity to pollute the soul, sexual ethics, according to Jehovanist ideology, must
emphasize the need to suppress sexual desire except for the purposes of
procreation which is the only absolutely necessary and therefore justifiable
purpose of sexual expression. All other sexual acts and desires were deemed
immoral. According to Don Ward (1971),

> These standards, as they originally evolved, reflected the need to tie
> sexual activity to procreation. Any use of sex that did not contribute
> to reproduction was lustful, even immoral. This emphasis on procrea-
> tion in time gave rise to the moral restrictions against homosexuality,
> masturbation, and the use of contraceptives: they impeded or pre-
> vented procreation. (p. 205)

Mosher (1992) suggests that the doctrines of Thomas Aquinas, another of
Christianity's more influential theologians, express the Jehovanist ideological construction of sexual morality.

> Aquinas expounded an eight-fold truth: (1) seminal discharge defines
> the essence of sexual intercourse, (2) the only moral function of sexual
> intercourse is procreation, (3) the act of procreation is completed only
> when the child becomes an adult, (4) procreators are obligated to
> provide for their issue until adulthood, (5) an unadulterous monoga-
> mous marriage is the best environment for socializing and moralizing
> children, (6) females are inferior to males, (7) male acts as the female's
> governor in marriage, and (8) divorce is improper. Thus, the only
> moral sex is coitus in the missionary position between marital partners
> for the purposes of procreation, experienced without too much pleas-
> ure, passion or affection. (Mosher, 1992, p. 21)

While Jehovanist sexual ideology has a long history, rooted in theological interpretations of human nature and sexuality, its taboo-ridden conceptualization of sexuality continues to express itself, often in nonreligious
terms, in contemporary society. "Although Jehovanism proper has produced no original argument against sex since Kant, its critical thrust has

continued in other forms. We may label 'Neo-Jehovanist' those utterances that express the antisexual impulse euphemistically without acknowledging its religious inspiration" (Davis, 1983, p. 171). According to Davis (1983) the influence of an implicitly Jehovanist sexual ideology is evident in the expression of "a theory of concomitant evil to convince those who do not find illicit sex despicable in itself that they should at least find deplorable the biological, psychological, and social evils that necessarily accompany it" (p. 207). Thus Neo-Jehovanists

> have claimed that premarital sex ("sexual freedom", "the new moral-ity") leads to "insecurity and hurt" and "dashed expectations" as well as "emotional problems" including "depression", "neurotic behavior", and "feelings of inadequacy", not to mention "loss of appetite" and "headaches." (Davis, 1983, p. 209)

Not surprisingly, from this perspective, adolescent sexual activity is not just immoral in the theological sense, but given its consequences it cannot be rationally justified.

> Jehovanist social psychologists often accuse teenagers who engage in premarital sex of giving in to "peer pressure." This accusation assumes not only that no adolescent who concluded that the benefits of sexual activity outweigh its detriments could be rational, but also that their own opinion of adolescent sex is completely uninfluenced by the "peer pressure" of their own colleagues. (Davis, 1983, p. 210)

As we shall see in Chapter Three, this Jehovanist perspective on adolescent sexuality permeates many contemporary sexuality education programs in the schools.

In sum, Jehovanist sexual ideology is restrictive in that heterosexual intercourse within marriage is seen as the only morally valid sexual behav-iour. All other sexual acts are, by nature, immoral. The moral codes of Jehovanist sexual ideology have constituted the core of Western sexual morality. All other ideological constructions have been conceived in terms of an oppositional relation to the central moral precepts of Jehovanist sexual ideology.

In analyzing the sexual politics of contemporary America, Seidman (1992) describes a struggle between "two broadly conceived sexual ideolo-gies" (p. 5): romanticism and libertarianism. According to Seidman (1992), "The conflict between these two sexual ideologies is at the core of many sexual and social struggles" (p. 6) and they "project antithetical sexual constructions" (p. 7). "The presence of these two sexual ideologies divides Americans on issues of homosexuality, teen sex, cohabitation, sex educa-tion, public sex, pornography etc. By and large the two sides remain polarized" (p. 178). Within this dualism of ideologies, Romanticism ex-presses an approach to human sexuality that is restrictive in nature.[1]

Seidman (1992) offers a typology of sexual ideology that is similar to but more complex than that proposed by Davis (1983). While the restrictive ethics of Jehovanism is rooted in a resolutely negative evaluation of sexual-ity, Romanticism, although highly suspicious of the sexual impulse, does see sexuality as a potentially positive force, provided that it is carefully control-led. While Romanticists leave open the possibility that sexual activity can be beneficial in terms of enhancing intimate relationships, they share with Jehovanists an emphasis on the dangers of sexual expression and the need for a restrictive sexual ethics. On the one hand, "The Romanticist believes that to harness the beneficial aspects of sex, eros must be connected to and kept intertwined with emotional, social and spiritual intimacies" (Seidman, 1992, p. 6). On the other hand, a liberalization of sexual norms is, to the Romanticist, not only unhealthy, but is a threat to social cohesion. "For them, the imagery of a sexual revolution evoked anticipations of libidinal chaos, the breakdown of family and moral order, and national crisis and social decline" (Seidman, 1992, p. 21). In sum, while Jehovanism sees only procreation as a positive outcome of sexual expression, Romanticism adds the idea that sexual expression can help build intimacy within a committed relationship. In this respect, although it takes a restrictive approach to sexual behaviour, Romanticism does have a sex-positive element.

However, in some fundamental ways, Jehovanism and Romanticism are synonymous. That is, Davis (1983) and Seidman (1992) are describing what seems to be the same ideological perspective. For example, according to Seidman (1992), those Romanticists who oppose homosexuality mirror Jehovanists "by appealing primarily to a Judeo-Christian religious tradition and a concept of natural law, both of which were said to be organized around a heterosexual familial order" (p. 177). In many respects, Romanticism reflects the Neo-Jehovanist tendency to rely on psycho-social, rather than theological, arguments to emphasize the potential evils of sexuality. So, for example, like the Neo-Jehovanist, the Romanticist rejects the possible validity of sex between teenagers "on the grounds that adolescents lack the maturity to approach sex in an intimate committed relationship" (Seidman, 1992, p. 6).

In historical perspective, the Romanticist view of sexuality clearly has its roots in the traditional Judeo-Christian conceptualization of sexuality as a force that, if not carefully controlled, could wreak havoc on the individual and society. Seidman (1992) cites Victorian culture as a prime example of Romanticist sexual ideology in practice.

> Many Victorians held that sexuality is an enormously powerful, life-giving-and-enhancing force that must be expressed. Yet, they were equally convinced that sexual expression automatically elicits lust, which carries serious personal and social dangers. The Victorians responded to this dilemma by organizing an intimate culture that attempted to control and spiritualize lust or sublimate it into productive social projects. Sexual expression was legitimated only within a heterosexual, coitus centered, marital norm. As the campaigns against masturbation and the moral reform efforts to spiritualize sex and marriage indicate, Victorian intimate culture sought to affirm sex expression while purging it of its carnal aspects. (p. 24)

With this Romanticist sexual ideology, the Victorians repudiated the subversive ideas popularized by the infamous eighteenth-century thinker the Marquis de Sade who

> insisted that physical and spiritual passion need have little to do with one another. Sade was the arch anti-Romantic when, in the novel *Juliette*, he asked, "Can't you go to bed with a woman without loving her, and can't you love her without going to bed with her?" (Robinson, 1976, p. 194)

Seidman (1992) goes on to say that in seeking to relieve sex of its nefarious aspects, the Romanticist ideology "promoted a politics of sexual restriction. It sought to limit sexual choice by severely circumscribing the socially available opportunities for sexual expression and by stigmatizing nonconventional sexual expression" (p. 24).

During the 20th century, however, particularly during the 1960s and 1970s, the influence of Romanticist sexual ideology waned as more permissive approaches to sexuality began to inform social attitudes and sexual behaviour. This decline in the influence of Romanticist sexual ideology is readily seen in the evolution of sexual attitudes from the 1950s to the 1970s. For example, Romanticism encourages sexual activity only within committed heterosexual relationships, particularly marriage. This Romanticist norm of acceptable sexual behaviour was widely endorsed, especially for women, during the 1950s. At that time only 14-17% of women believed that it was acceptable for females to engage in premarital sex. By the 1960s the number had jumped to 45% and in 1973, 87% believed that it was acceptable for women to engage in premarital sex (Allgeier & Allgeier, 1988, p. 424). Large-scale introduction of the birth control pill during the 1960s helped launch the "sexual revolution" by allowing women, particularly those who were young and unmarried, to partake of the pleasures of intercourse without the threat of unwanted pregnancy. The pill enabled people to rid themselves of one of the major negative consequences of sexual expression. In an age where premarital sexual activity carried the risk of both moral condemnation and the practical consequences of an unwanted pregnancy, the moral dictates of Romanticism were more difficult to reject. When birth control enabled people to eliminate a major consequence of sexual behaviour, the foundation of Romanticist sexual ideology had lost one of its critical supports, leading many people to reject its restrictive approach to sexual behaviour.

However, as Seidman (1992) notes, the sexual ideology of Romanticism has enjoyed a considerable resurgence during the 1980s and 1990s. The increasing popularity of restrictive approaches to sexuality grew out of a dissatisfaction with the perceived outcomes of the sexual permissiveness of the 1960s and 1970s: skyrocketing divorce rates, single motherhood, teen pregnancy, abortion, rising STD rates, and AIDS. In addition, increasing permissiveness was seen to contribute to emotional alienation and disturbances.

> Psychologists spoke of a rising tide of anxieties associated with sexual performance, impotence, and loneliness; feminists highlighted an epidemic of child abuse and violence towards women stemming, in part, from an intimate culture encouraging the objectification of individuals as mere bodies to be exploited for personal pleasure and adventure. Cultural critics assailed American intimate conventions for promoting emotionally shallow and callous behavior, and for reducing individuals to mere bodies and organs. Many Americans thought the source of this malaise to be liberationist ideology that was characterized as excessively permissive, that placed too much value on erotic pleasure, and that was so tolerant toward variant sexual expressions that it undermined moral standards. (Seidman, 1992, p. 64)

Seidman (1992) associates the re-emergence of Romanticist sexual ideology with the rise of the social values and politics of the "New Right," "a loose coalition of political, religious, and single-issue pro-life and pro-family groups which combined grass-roots mobilization with professional lobbying" (p. 70). Generally speaking, the New Right has sought to strengthen "family values" by advocating sexual ethics aimed at restoring the supremacy of the patriarchal nuclear family. This involved strenuous opposition to abortion, pornography, the feminist movement, homosexual rights, and premarital sex. In terms of teen sexuality, one of the primary achievements of the New Right was the passage in the United States Congress of the Adolescent Family Life Act in 1981. The Act stipulated that federal government funds would only go towards sexuality education programs that promoted premarital sexual abstinence. The Act also prohibited agencies that "advocate, promote, or encourage abortion" from receiving government funding (Bruess & Greenberg, 1994, p. 164). According to Reiss (1990) the Adolescent Family Life Act reflected a "dogmatic, sexually restrictive approach" and was evidence of a bubbling to the surface of a "residual Victorianism." More recently, a 1996 welfare reform bill has provided for $50 million in U.S. federal funding for abstinence-only sexuality education. As I shall discuss further in Chapter Three, this legislation reflects an attempt to impose a sexual ideology on today's youth.

It is significant to note that Seidman (1992) places Radical feminism within the Romanticist camp. At first glance this may seem puzzling because it aligns social-political conservatives with the most provocative segment of the feminist movement. When we think of the conflict between Restrictive and Permissive sexual ideology in terms of the traditional dichotomy between conservative and liberal, it is, on the surface, natural to place the feminist movement within the Liberal-Permissive spectrum of ideological beliefs. However, as is often noted, there exists considerable diversity in feminist positions on sexuality. Most observers have cast these differences in terms of the sometimes conflicting points of view expressed by Radical as opposed to Liberal feminists (e.g., McCormick, 1994). While there are, in turn, differences within the overall Radical and Liberal feminist positions, Seidman (1992) suggests that the sexual perspectives of many Radical feminists fall within the scope of Romanticist sexual ideology. For these feminists,

The sex act itself should exhibit intimate qualities by being gentle, nurturing, tender and person-oriented. Sex that occurs outside an intimate setting or sex that occurs within a loving relationship but that is centered on bodily, sensual pleasure is morally degrading and unacceptable. (p. 106)

Because these quite specific criteria are applied to the moral evaluation of the sex act, some Radical feminists have been accused of "promulgating a restrictive sexual ethic that reinforces a politic of sexual repression." (Ibid.)

Radical feminism is defined, first and foremost, in terms of its political theory, by its delineation of the structures of male domination which are seen to be inherent and pervasive in human societies, and by its goal to dismantle these structures (Jagger, 1983). This, in and of itself, does not translate into a Restrictive sexual ethics. However, as evidenced in the work of some Radical feminists, this political programme, in some cases, includes a critique of sexual ethics that emphasizes the importance of allowing individuals to exercise free choice in making sexual decisions. For some feminists, the ethical and political project of making freedom of choice the raison d'être of the feminist movement unduly ignores the fact that within the context of a patriarchal society, extending the range of ethically approved sexual behaviours serves mainly to create new opportunities for men to oppress women. In sum, limiting the sexual choices available, a hallmark of Restrictive sexual ideology, is, in some Radical feminist perspectives, necessary in order to protect women from oppression.

A Romanticist perspective toward sex can be found in some prominent Radical feminist writings on sexuality. For example, Sheila Jeffreys' (1990) Radical feminist analysis of the sexual revolution of the 1960s and 1970s suggests not only that sexual liberalism is synonymous with moral relativism but also that the sexual revolution was "...really an exercise in training women to become experts in sexually servicing men, and to get over their own tastes and interests in order to become efficient at this task" (p. 110). By focussing on aspects of sexuality such as orgasmic potential and other, often unconventional, means of enhancing physical pleasure, the sexual revolution has further removed female sexuality from a world where sex, equality, nurture, and intimacy all go hand in hand. Here, we can see that the sentiment is Romanticist in nature because it limits the range of potentially positive outcomes of sexual activity to those which enhance, with a Radical feminist twist, the Romanticist ideal of mature intimate relationships.

This particular feminist approach to sexuality implies a restrictive sexual ethics in two fundamental ways. First, as other feminists, with a different perspective, have noted, from some Radical feminist perspectives,

> sex has to occur in a certain way for it to be good. And the only legitimate sex is very limited. It's not focused on orgasms, it's very gentle and it takes place in the context of a long-term, caring relationship. It's the missionary position of the women's movement. (English, Hollibaugh, & Rubin, 1987, p. 70)

Secondly, because some Radical feminists consider male sexual desire to be dependant on the sexual subordination of women, heterosexual sexual activity is seen as inherently immoral (Dworkin, 1987; MacKinnon, 1987; Jeffreys, 1990). If this is so, then, as Jefferys (1990) argues, "The demolition of heterosexual desire is a necessary step on the route to women's liberation" (p. 312). If heterosexual sexual interaction is, in the context of contemporary society, immoral, then it is evident that this Radical feminist approach to sexuality is Restrictive in that only very specific forms of sexual activity are permissable. All heterosexual acts that take place within the context of our male dominated society are morally suspect. The preference for homosexuality, lesbian sex in particular, does put Radical feminist thought at odds with what we might call mainstream Romanticism which generally opposes homosexuality. Radical feminism is, in some cases, however, appropriately described as Romanticist because it only affirms sexual acts with particular "intimate qualities."

Some Radical feminist approaches to the issue of pornography are illustrative of Restrictive ideological leanings and their subsequent union with the forces of political conservatism. For example, as Stanton (1992) points out,

> the feminist activism that led to the redefinition of pornography as violence against women c. 1975, rather than the "liberal" view of healthy sexual expression against a puritanical society, influenced and gained support from the 1986 Meese commission that pornography is and causes violence. Some feminists—notably Women against Pornography—formed an alliance with the New Right to ban sexually explicit materials: the ordinance written by Andrea Dworkin and Catherine A. MacKinnon, though subsequently overturned, declared pornography a violation of women's civil rights. While it aimed to combat misogyny, this alliance also supported broad conservative goals

of imposing stringent limitations on sexual practices and discourses. (p. 13)

It would certainly be an overgeneralization to suggest that all people who consider themselves to be Radical feminists hold a Restrictive sexual ideology. One cannot, by definition, be equated with the other. Nor does one necessarily imply the other. However, the propensity for some Radical feminists to endorse sometimes fairly strict limitations on what counts as acceptable sexual behaviour does support Seidman's (1992) argument that some Radical feminists hold a Romanticist sexual ideology. This becomes particularly evident when Radical feminists are compared to Liberal feminists who typically place a greater emphasis on increasing the choices available to women in all spheres of life.

In sum, Romanticist sexual ideology falls squarely into the Restrictive camp. On one hand, it acknowledges only a very narrow range of beneficial outcomes that can result from sexual activity. On the other hand, Romanticists grant moral approval only to sexual behaviour that takes place within a very specific context. With the exception of the Radical feminist perspective, all sexual acts that fall outside of the context of the heterosexual, coitus centred, marital norm, even if they are subject to mutual consent and pleasure, are deemed immoral. So, for example, by most Romanticist ethical criteria, a sexual interaction between two homosexual adolescents must be, in and of itself, immoral. Homosexuality does not conform to the coitus centred, marital norm. In this respect it threatens a social order based on the nuclear family. Just as importantly, according to the Romanticist view, adolescents are incapable of mature committed relationships and therefore their sex acts can have no legitimate moral purpose. Thus, Romanticism, like Jehovanism, is not only restrictive in its approach to sexual ethics, its inflexibility in judging the validity of specific sexual acts adds to Romanticism and Jehovanism an element of moral absolutism. Moral absolutism, as we shall now see, tends to be a central feature of Restrictive sexual ideology.

Jeffrey Weeks (1985; 1986) describes three different approaches which he suggests have influenced our thinking about sexuality in Western culture: the Absolutist, Liberal, and Libertarian. Although Weeks (1985) employs the term "approaches" rather than ideology, he is referring to "strategies for the regulation and control of sexuality" (p. 52). "Each of these evokes different assumptions about the true meaning of sex" (Weeks, 1985, p. 53). Or put another way, "What we believe sex is, or ought to be, structures our responses to it" (Weeks, 1986, p. 100). In these respects, the approaches described by Weeks constitute ideologies. Weeks' descriptions of these approaches are particularly useful because his differentiation between the Absolutist and Liberal approaches, in particular, provides a basis for a more precise analysis of the sexual ethics inherent in the broader Restrictive and Permissive ideological categories.

Of the three dominant approaches described by Weeks, the Absolutist clearly represents a restrictive ideological approach to sexuality. In essence, with the Absolutist approach, Weeks is describing a perspective that is reflective of the Jehovanist and Romanticist sexual ideologies.

> Historically, we are heirs of the absolutist tradition. This has been based on a fundamental belief that the disruptive powers of sex can only be controlled by a clear-cut morality, intricately embedded in a particular set of social institutions: marriage, heterosexuality, family life and (at least in the Judaic-Christian traditions), monogamy. This absolutist morality is deeply rooted in the Christian West, but through its grounding may be embraced as readily by the atheist as by the Christian (or other religious) who is ready to worship at the foot of strong, moral values. Moral absolutism has deeply influenced our general culture, and in particular the forms of legal regulation, many of which still survive. (Weeks, 1986, p. 100)

The convergence of moral absolutism with Jehovanist sexual ideology is relatively straight forward. They are both rooted in an Aristotelian fixed view of human nature that has served as a foundation of the traditional Judeo-Christian moral perspective. Central to this view is the notion that "human beings were created by God as unchanging archetypes, thus determining standards of human behavior for all time" (Francoeur, 1987, p. 3). This world view developed out of rationalistic and theological presuppositions regarding the orderliness of nature including the idea that human nature is the work of a divine architect and is revealed through reason and divine revelation. The physical world and human nature are viewed as being governed by fixed and immutable laws. According to Mosher (1989), from this perspective moral principles are expressed

> as authority-given rules such as the Ten Commandments. People with a conventional form of moral judgement believe moral rules were fixed forever on Mount Sinai. Not only are God-given rules everlasting, but they are always enforced. (p. 496)

Thus, a major underlying assumption of this ideology is that "...these moral regulations apply basically for all times, all societies, all cultures, all age groups, and all individuals alike" (Guindon, 1986, p. 5).

In the realm of sexuality, the early Christian scholars deemed certain sexual behaviours (i.e. procreative intercourse) as natural, and therefore morally permissible, while others were deemed as unnatural (i.e., masturbation, sodomy), and therefore immoral. As the overwhelmingly dominant moral authorities of the time, these theologians took on the responsibility of setting the standard of morally acceptable sexual behaviour and in turn determined the sexual moral norms of Western society. In effect, "responsibility for wise-decision-making in sexual matters was transferred, one way or another to an exterior authoritative agency" (Guindon, 1986, p. 3).

We can see that this perspective is absolutist in the sense that once the moral rules of sexual behaviour have been established they are, like the Ten Commandments, etched in stone. They are unchangeable and not subject to modification. This approach is also clearly restrictive in nature in that it is highly proscriptive in terms of what specific forms of sexual behaviour are morally valid.

One of the central features of the moral absolutist approach is that it focusses on specific sexual acts as the object of moral evaluation. Jehovanist sexual ideology employs an act-centred focus to conceptualize the process of sexual ethics. In their discussion of the traditional Catholic moral evaluation of sexual conduct Kosnick, Carroll, Cunningham, Modras, and Schulte (1977) succinctly summarize this act-centred sexual ethics.

> Catholic tradition in evaluating moral behavior has placed a heavy emphasis in recent centuries on the objective moral nature of the given act itself. Particularly with regard to sexuality, it was believed that there is a meaning intrinsic to the very nature of the act itself—a meaning that is absolutely unchangeable and in no way modifiable by extenuating circumstances or special context. Thus, masturbation, any premarital sexual pleasure, adultery, fornication, homosexuality, sodomy, and bestiality were considered intrinsically evil acts, seriously immoral, and under no circumstances justifiable. This approach was influenced to a great extent by an oversimplification of the natural law theory of St. Thomas, the negative sin-oriented approach of the moral manuals, and a strong desire for clear, precise absolute norms to govern moral conduct. (p. 88)

Consequently, Jehovanist sexual ideology has a simple, straightforward moral code. A specific, and very narrow set of sexual behaviours are morally acceptable: all others, are not.

Romanticist sexual ideology is also absolutist by virtue of its act-centred approach, although it slightly expands the context under which morally acceptable sexual activity can take place. With the exception of the Romanticist element within Radical Feminism, sexual behaviour can achieve moral validity, in the Romanticist view, if, and only if, it enhances emotional intimacy within mature, monogamous, heterosexual marriage. So, for example, while Jehovanism condemns adolescent sexual behaviour on the basis of God-given moral dictates, Romanticism rejects the behaviour on the grounds that teenagers are too immature to be involved in emotionally sound, stable relationships. Both ideologies take an absolutist approach to adolescent sex because they disapprove of the behaviour under any circumstances and with no exceptions. Once these arguments have been established as ideologically constructed "facts," either by theologians or psychologists, there is no need for individuals to contemplate alternatives or engage in moral deliberation: the path to morally valid behaviour is self-evident and must be followed with faith and discipline.

In sum, Restrictive sexual ideology traces its origins to a fixed view of human nature that emerged as a fundamental component of the early Christian tradition's understanding of the universe. If human nature is a fixed, divinely inspired creation, moral truth is, objectively speaking, available to us through divine revelation. As we have seen, Augustine was an exemplar of this world view with his belief that "absolute or objective knowledge of the good was obtainable through direct mystical experience of the divinely revealed truth of God" (Kurtines & Gewirtz, 1984, p. 12). Since this truth was derived from a God in the heavens, unaffected by changes in the earthly human social world, its substance was unalterable.

Until the age of "enlightenment," beginning in the seventeenth century, this fixed conception of human nature and morality held an almost total monopoly of belief in Western culture.

> Since the fifth century A.D., the intellectual history of the West had been unified by an unshakable faith in the truth of the Christian revelation and an equally deep and abiding belief that reason (guided by faith) would ultimately provide objective or certain knowledge about the world. Consequently, for very long in the intellectual history

of the Western world, questions of morality did not seem truly problematic. Issues were raised; differences encountered; fine points debated. But never did it appear that issues could not be settled, that
differences could not be resolved within a larger, commonly accepted
framework. The Western world experienced a unity of thought like
never before and perhaps never again. This unity of thought provided
an ethic or morality. (Kurtines & Gewirtz, 1984, pp. 14-15)

Combined with a negative conceptualization of the nature of human
sexuality—the belief that sex is essentially dirty and sinful—the principles
of morality inherent in this unity of thought yielded the absolutist act-centred sexual ethics that characterizes Restrictive sexual ideology.

These are the key components of Restrictive sexual ideology, and, as I
will show in Chapter Three, many contemporary forms of sexuality education in the schools take their cue from these ideas.

Permissive Sexual Ideology

Until relatively recently, Restrictive sexual ideology, particularly the
religiously inspired doctrines of Jehovanism, held a near monopoly on the
sexual moral discourse of Western society. A number of factors, including
demographic, scientific, and philosophical transformations, have fundamentally changed the nature of society, and in the process produced
alternative ideological perspectives which have arisen to challenge the
supremacy of Restrictive sexual ideology. These, relatively more recent,
ideological perspectives share a fundamental premise that sexuality, rather
than being a primarily negative force requiring strict control, is either benign
or positive in its ability to provide pleasure and contribute to self-fulfilment
and psychological adjustment. As opposed to seeing the need to limit the
context and range of morally acceptable sexual behaviours, these ideological
perspectives suggest that the human condition, both at the individual and
societal level, is better served by a sexual ethics that replaces Absolutist,
act-centred evaluations of sexual conduct with methods of moral evaluation
that emphasize individual differences in desire and person-centred relational concerns such as mutual consent, pleasure, and respect. Within such
a framework, the range of morally acceptable sexual behaviours is greatly
expanded. Ideological perspectives of this kind are clearly more permissive
in nature than the Restrictive sexual ideology.

A key factor in the emergence of Permissive sexual ideology is a historical trend away from the theologically rooted fixed view of human nature which was the genesis of Restrictive sexual ideology. This historical trend towards secularized, evolutionary conceptualizations of human nature, particularly in the last several hundred years, has dramatically reshaped the intellectual, social-political climate of Western culture. As Francoeur (1987) puts it, "no greater revolution has occurred in the history of human thought than the radical shift from a fixed world view rooted in unchanging archetypes to a dynamic, evolving world view based on populations and individuals" (p. 52).

The emergence of this alternative world view would have profound implications for the way we think about sexuality and its role in defining human nature. A concept of human nature that is dynamic rather than fixed, evolutionary rather than theological, creates the conditions for a Permissive sexual ideology that Davis (1983) labels *Naturalism*.[2] Naturalist sexual ideology, according to Davis (1983) is characterized by "its connection with a broader historical tradition that interprets sexual phenomena in terms of nature rather than in terms of the sacred" (p. 183).

> Modern Naturalism is the heir of several historical trends, which have given its conception of copulation a distinct character. Like many formerly sacred activities, sex has been caught up in the process of secularization, which has severed its spiritual ties. Naturalist metaphysics is that sex has no metaphysics. Sex has none of the tremendous cosmic meaning for modern Naturalists that it has for Jehovanists. (Davis, 1983, p. 185)

The removal of sexuality from the realm of the sacred is important for several reasons. First, and perhaps most importantly, such a move makes possible a clean break with the tradition of looking at sexuality as something that is necessarily, or has a great potential to be, a corrupting presence. If sexuality is, like human beings themselves, just another part of nature, it can be more easily viewed as either harmless, neutral, or potentially beneficial. This Naturalist ideology takes a dim view of restrictive approaches not only because of their behavioural restrictions, but also because they instill feelings of guilt and shame which smother and stunt the beneficial aspects of sexuality. Freeing sexuality from religiously inspired guilt and shame has been one of the primary political projects of Naturalist sexual ideology. While theology was the vehicle for propounding Jehovanist sexual ideology, the modern sciences of biology and psychology provided Naturalist sexual ideology with its sex positive or sex neutral world view. Davis (1983) cites Havelock Ellis, Sigmund Freud, Alfred Kinsey, and Masters and Johnson as examples of the modern sexologists who have treated sex from a Naturalist ideological perspective. Robinson (1976) refers to the rise of this alternative sexual paradigm as the "modernization of sex." According to Robinson (1976), Alfred Kinsey, who conducted and published the first large scale surveys of American sexual behaviour in the 1940s and 1950s, is a pivotal figure in the growth of the modern view of sexuality. Robinson's (1976) characterization of Kinsey reveals that the famous sexologist was not only anti-Jehovanist in his belief that sexuality was benevolent, but also anti-Romanticist in his view that sex need not be tied to emotional intimacy.

> He is not so unqualified a sexual materialist as was the Marquis de Sade, but he sought above all else to separate human sexual experience from its elaborate emotional associations. Those associations, he believed, placed unnecessary restrictions on the expression of an innocent physical need. Only when repressed did sexual urges threaten emotional stability, and thus a rational society, he implied, would seek to promote not only a positive but an essentially casual attitude toward sexuality. The notion that sex was permissible only when persons truly loved one another was to him no less absurd than the belief that masturbation caused insanity. (Robinson, 1977, p. 194)

A fundamental aspect of Naturalist sexual ideology is its opposition to Jehovanism's hostility toward sexuality.

> Naturalists are divided between moderates who tolerate sex, and radicals, who venerate it. Moderate Naturalists find most forms of sex "not harmful"; radical Naturalists find them actually beneficial, particularly for mental health. (Davis, 1983, p. 185)

The second major implication of Naturalism's removal of sexuality from the realm of the sacred is to take matters of sexual morality out of the hands of God, and by extension the theological authorities, and place such questions in the hands of individuals. If sexuality is no longer viewed as a potent corrupter of the spirit, but is alternatively seen as a natural biological function, albeit one that retains considerable social and moral significance, the foundation of sexual ethics is subject to modification.

The Naturalist's ethics for human sexuality are the same ethics of concern and respect for persons that he or she applies to all human interactions. The Humanistic spirit of the sexual Naturalist favors freedom of sexual choice and compassionate respect for others' sexual choices. The Naturalist respects each of us as an end, because each of us is a *person* with moral autonomy. Humanistic respect for persons translates into Naturalist respect for people's rights to make their own sexual choices. Sexuality—neither idealized nor demonized by the Naturalist—becomes a natural part of living. (Mosher, 1989, pp. 493-494)

With his tripartite typology of approaches to the regulation of sexuality, Weeks (1985; 1986) contrasts the restrictive Absolutist approach with what he calls the Liberal and Libertarian approaches. In essence, the Liberal and Libertarian approaches to sexual regulation described by Weeks (1985; 1986) are the applied ethics of Davis' (1983) moderate Naturalists and radical Naturalists. I have argued that there is a logical relationship between theoretical assumptions about the nature of sexuality and the complementary system of ethics that is adopted to regulate sexual behaviour. An examination of Weeks' (1985; 1986) descriptions of the Liberal and Libertarian approaches to the regulation of sexuality provides further insights into the sexual ethics of Naturalist sexual ideology in particular and Permissive sexual ideology in general.

The Libertarian approach to the regulation of sexual behaviour is at the perimeter of the permissive end of the continuum of sexual ideologies. It celebrates sex as a subversive means of disrupting the social order. Weeks (1986) cites the Marquis de Sade, George Bataille, Jean Genet, Wilhelm Reich and Herbert Marcuse as representative of the Libertarian approach. This approach has an explicitly political agenda. The more transgressive a sexual act is, the more likely that the more radical of the libertarians will give it their moral approval.

> At the heart of this approach is the belief that sexual repression is essential to social oppression; and that the moment of social sexual liberation should necessarily coincide with the moment of social revolution. It is a utopian and millenarian project, and that has been its major source of energy. (Weeks, 1985, p. 55)

While some conservatives have accused contemporary sexuality educators of holding this kind of libertarian sexual ideology, and although the Libertarian approach has had some influence on the sexual politics of the

Western world, particularly in the 1960s, theoretical perspectives focussing on the political ramifications of the social organization of sexuality have not been a major influence on contemporary sexuality education programs (Carlson, 1992).

With his categorization of the Liberal approach to the regulation of sexuality, Weeks (1985; 1986) is describing what has become, along with moral absolutism, one of the two most influential moral frameworks for evaluating sexual conduct. The theoretical points of departure of the Liberal approach to sexual ethics are secular moral concepts such as individual rights and moral autonomy and distinctions between morality and law. From this perspective, "The duty of law is to regulate public order and to maintain acceptable (though by implication changing) standards of public decency, not to patrol personal life" (Weeks, 1986, p. 54). From the legal standpoint,

> The two classic propositions on which this approach relies are derived from John Stuart Mill: that no conduct should be interfered with unless it involves harm to others; and that it is not the law's business to enforce morals. The assumption is that intervention should only be contemplated if the harm caused by it will be less than the damage caused by the continuation of a given condition. (Weeks, 1985, p. 215)

This combined focus on individual rights and utilitarian concepts of social regulation have underlined legal perspectives that have challenged, mainly in the last several decades, sexual laws based on traditional, usually Christian absolutist, concepts of sexual morality. Indeed, it is in this way that we can speak of the "liberalization" of laws pertaining to sexuality. In those jurisdictions where sex laws have been relaxed or liberalized, these changes have been justified on the grounds that the state does not belong in the bedrooms of its citizens so long as the behaviours in question do not infringe on the rights of others and do not have a demonstrated harm to society. According to Weeks (1985), this distinction between law and morality "has been an important strategy in undermining the absolutist approach, and in creating certain spaces for greater individual freedom" (p. 54).

It is here, in the arena of an individual's sexual morality, that the disagreements between divergent ideological perspectives are most divisive. The Liberal approach stands in stark contrast to the Absolutist approach. Whereas the Absolutist approach relies on a universalized, fixed evaluation of specific sexual acts, implying a socialization process and sexual ethics based on the acceptance of doctrine, the Liberal approach demands individual moral deliberation based on personal choice, context, and needs, and secular moral principles such as equality, justice, and so on. Generally speaking, Liberal philosophy places a "...reliance on individual judgement, uncoerced and unindoctrinated, rather than on established authority in determining matters of truth and morality" (Jagger, 1983, p. 33).

The centrality, within the Liberal approach to sexual ethics, of individual choice and context places individual deliberation, rather than specific sexual acts, at the pinnacle of moral evaluation. This results in what may be designated as person-centred sexual ethics.

> The person is considered as an essentially free being with a capacity for reason, love, and compassion, and the potential for becoming more authentically his or her human self. Sexuality is proposed as an integral aspect of a multifaceted person; sexual relating as an expression of the person in all his or her complexity; and sexual ethics as a specific application of person-centered as opposed to more legalistic act-centered ethics. In making decisions and judgements using this approach, the person-in-context is considered rather than simply judging an act in and of itself as ethically right or wrong. Answering the reality-revealing questions of who, what, where, when, why, and how, as well as considering the viable alternatives to and the foreseeable effects of an act, enables participants to make informed decisions and judgements. The task is to discern the values, choices, and actions that enhance the essential and sacred humanness of the person(s) involved. (Lawlor, Morris, McKay, Purcell, & Comeau, 1990, p. 10)

While this person-centred approach, with its focus on individual deliberation with respect to making sexual choices, is more permissive than restrictive in nature, it does suggest that sexual behaviour does need to be guided by moral principles derived from the Liberal philosophical tradition. For example, in rejecting Absolutist sexual ethics and endorsing sexual pluralism, Reiss (1992) proposes that sexual decision making should be guided by the moral principles of honesty, equality, and responsibility.

> To oppose sexual dogmatism is not to favor an "anything goes," libertine philosophy. If we oppose the prohibition of alcohol, that does not mean we favor drunkenness. A person can be sexually tolerant and still be discriminating. To favor a rational, thinking, and caring approach to sexual choices is the way to bring control into our sexual lives. The pluralistic position explicitly requires moral restraint by its

insistence that we seek to be honest, equal, and responsible in *all* our sexual relationships. Pluralism is surely not saying "just say yes." If there were a slogan for pluralism, it would be: "choose wisely." (Reiss, 1992, p. 219)

This person-centred approach to sexual ethics has featured prominently in Permissive ideological conceptualizations of sexuality education in the schools. As Weeks (1986) suggests, "To Liberals, sexuality education was the only means of spreading the information on which rational choices could be made" (p. 95).

Seidman's (1992) conceptualization of Libertarian sexual ideology generally encompasses Davis' (1983) Naturalist and Weeks' (1985; 1986) Liberal categories. [Sexuality is seen in a positive light and is evaluated in terms of its ability to bring happiness.] *but only temporary.*

Sex is viewed as a positive, beneficial, joyous phenomenon. Its expression is connected to personal health, happiness, self-fulfilment, and social progress. Sex is said to have multiple meanings; it can be justified as an act of self expression or pleasure, a sign of affection, love or a procreative act. Sexual expression is said to be legitimate in virtually all adult consensual social exchanges, although most libertarians place sex in a romantic, loving bond at the top of their value hierarchy. (Seidman, 1992, pp. 5-6)

In characterizing the sexual ethics of this ideology, Seidman (1992) suggests that Libertarians reject absolutist act-centred evaluations of sexual conduct and bring "a highly individualistic liberal concept of free choice to legitimate practices" (Seidman, 1992, p. 206).

Libertarians aim to defend "benign sexual variation" by abandoning a morality centered on the intrinsic moral nature of sex acts. They aim to expand legitimate sexual expression or to reduce state and social controls, by advocating for a minimalistic ethic: sexual exchanges acquire legitimacy to the extent that they are mutually consensual and perhaps entail mutual pleasure and affection. (Seidman, 1992, pp. 205-206)

In their position on teen sexuality, Libertarians mirror the view of Naturalists and Liberals in that they "would generally defend, at least in principle, sex between adolescents if it were consensual and responsible (e.g., involved contraceptives)" (Seidman, 1992, p. 6).

If some forms of Radical feminism fall within the scope of Romanticism, its main rival within the spectrum of feminist thought, Liberal feminism, fits within the parameters of Seidman's category of Libertarianism. In terms of sexuality, the Liberal feminist project is to expand women's sexual self-determination so that it is on a level playing field with that of men. "Liberal feminists seek to remove any restrictions interfering with women's sexual autonomy and gratification, those imposed by men and those imposed by other women" (McCormick, 1994, p. 9). So while Radical feminism would substitute the restrictions placed on female sexuality by patriarchy with a new set of restrictions, Liberal feminists seek to move from patriarchal restrictions to greater female sexual autonomy without defining the specific characteristics of what constitutes acceptable sexual behaviour. Rather, "they formulate their critique of contemporary sexual norms in terms of their characteristic values of equality, liberty, and justice" (Jagger, 1983, p. 178). This is clearly a Permissive ideological approach to sexuality in that it calls for greater sexual freedom for women and it is up to women as individuals to decide where this freedom will take them. As Seidman (1992) notes, "many women will, and indeed have, repudiated a sexual ideology that stipulates that sex is legitimate only as an expression of love, only as enacted in acts of personal tenderness and only if confined to long-term relationships" (p. 130). Finally, Liberal feminism reflects Permissive sexual ideology in that it sees the essence of human sexuality as positive in nature. Indeed, affirming women's right to self-determined sexual pleasure is seen by many Liberal feminists as an integral component of the quest for full gender equality. For these feminists, the hope is that women will be "less compelled to approach sex as a domain of danger" (Seidman, 1992, p. 130).

As with all of the ideologies described in this chapter, Libertarians attach great importance to sexuality in so far as the conceptualization of its nature, purpose and the ethics employed to guide it have significant implications for social life in general. This can be seen in the Libertarian interpretation of the loosening of sexual norms during the 1960s and the subsequent roll back of these trends during the 1970s and 1980s.

> Libertarians describe the 1960s as a time of progress in which sex was supposedly liberated from restrictive control of the moral guardians of a repressive order. Sex was accepted as a sensual pleasure; eros moved out of the bedroom into the public arena, thereby losing some of its repressive mystique; tolerance for nonconventional sexual practices and lifestyles expanded. For many Libertarians, the late 1970s and

1980s is viewed as a time of reaction, even backlash. Sexual freedom and diversity are seen as under attack; eros is being blamed for social ills from AIDS to divorce. The forces of order and repression are said to be swelling as they have successfully linked, in the public mind, sexual freedom and permissiveness to social disorder and decline. (Seidman, 1992, pp. 6-7)

Davis' (1983) Naturalism, Weeks' (1985; 1986) Liberalism, and Seidman's (1992) Libertarianism are examples of Permissive sexual ideology. All three represent an opposition to the restrictive ideologies of Jehovanism, Absolutism, and Romanticism. These permissive ideologies are united by their positive view of sexuality and a person-centred sexual ethics which greatly expands the range of morally acceptable sexual activities. The rise of Permissive sexual ideology is the result of a number of historical trends including, most notably, the shift, within Western society, from a fixed to an evolutionary world view. What is problematic about all of this to Restrictive sexual ideologues, many of whom hold fixed, theistically oriented, world views, is that it allows human beings themselves to decide what is morally right and morally wrong.

The profound differences between the Restrictive and Permissive sexual ideologies in terms of the moral aspects of sexual behaviour can be illustrated through an uncomplicated example. An individual contemplating adultery (by adultery I mean the situation in which a married person engages in sexual activity with a person other than hi or her spouse) will follow very different paths of moral evaluation depending on whether he or she employs a Restrictive or Permissive ideological approach. From a Restrictive perspective the individual follows the biblical commandment "Thou Shall not commit adultery." From a Permissive perspective, for example Reiss' (1990) honesty, equality, responsibility approach, the issue is not so clear cut. The individual contemplating the act must decide through moral deliberation if, in this particular case, the act of adulterous sex will exhibit the qualities of honesty, equality, and responsibility with respect to all parties involved. The answer to this question is not self-evident but must be arrived at through the deliberative process. This example illustrates two very different approaches to sexual morality, each with a well established history.

Conclusion

In the first chapter we saw that the regulation of sexual behaviour is universally regarded as being a crucial factor in determining the nature of society. Western culture is, however, deeply divided on the wide range of issues relevant to the conceptualization and structuring of sexuality in our society. The Western cultural discourse on sexuality is characterized by a struggle between what I have called Restrictive and Permissive sexual ideologies. These ideologies represent diametrically opposed, yet internally consistent, beliefs about the nature and purpose of sexuality in human life and society. The struggle between the Restrictive and Permissive sexual ideologies is frequently seen as a battle for the soul of society itself.

> Today the permissives and the conservatives are organized for the politics of sex. The battlegrounds are abortion, legitimation of homosexuality, sex education in the schools, contraceptives for adolescents, AIDS, and sex research. Pat Buchanan, in his preoccupation with the homosexual menace, thinks this amounts to a war. But right now it is politics as usual. (Udry, 1993, p. 104)

Not surprisingly, the proponents of each of these ideologies have a keen interest in the nature and content of sexuality education in the schools. As a fundamental agent of socialization, the public school now plays a role in teaching youth about sexuality. Like the broader social disputes around sexuality, the controversy over sexuality education shows no signs of abating. Sexuality education has become a focal point in a larger ideological struggle between opposing views of sexuality.

Notes

1. Seidman's application of the label *Romanticist* to this particular brand of sexual ideology may seem curious to some readers. Romanticism is a term loosely applied to 18th and 19th century artistic and literary movements. There is a wide variety of interpretations of the meaning of Romanticism, although it may be said that most of the various strains of Romanticism are united by their opposition to classicism. In philosophy, Romanticism is most often associated with Jean Jacques Rousseau who professed a belief in the natural goodness of humanity. In my reading, it is likely that Seidman has chosen the term *Romanticism* to describe this sexual ideology because of its belief in the strong emotional bonding of mature relationships, which Romanticist sexual ideology holds in high regard. The emphasis is on intense emotion rather than reason or logic. This is congruent with the emphasis on emotions that is typical of much Romanticist thought.
2. The terms *Naturalism* and *Natural Law* are frequently used, particularly in philosophy. Although they both refer to aspects of *nature*, they have quite

different meanings. Naturalism, as a philosophy, generally refers to the position that all phenomena can be explained by means of natural, as opposed to supernatural, categories. In other words, natural science provides an over-all explanation of the universe. The theory of natural law, however, suggests that there are some basic and immutable laws that govern human nature. Moral principles flow from these laws. These laws are universal and unchangeable in that since they constitute *a priori* human nature, they are not subject to modification. Natural law has been particularly popular among Christian philosophers, whereas Naturalism lies at the root of empiricism. In these respects, Natural Law fits well with the fixed view of human nature characteristic of Restrictive sexual ideology and Naturalism is compatible with the secular, evolving world view of Permissive sexual ideology.

CHAPTER THREE

Sexual Ideology in the Schools

—··—··—··—··—··—··—··—··—··—··—··—.

"What masquerades as sex education is not education at all. It is selective propaganda which artificially encourages children to participate in adult sex, while it censors out the facts of life about the unhappy consequences. It is robbing children of their childhood."

(Schlafly, 1981)

"We have to reject the dogmatic sexual philosophy that states that it is always dangerous to encourage open discussion of sexuality with preadolescents....The way out of our sexual impasse is to reject traditional restraints on children's sexual education and to accept the importance of socializing our children to sexuality from birth onward."

(Reiss, 1990)

"The school is first and foremost an *educational* institution; as such its first duty must always be to teach children the truth and good values. The truth is that sexual activity by unmarried teenagers is harmful to them and harmful to society. The morally right value is for young people to avoid such activity."

(Lickona, 1991)

"...progressive educators must not abandon the field of school sexuality education to those who advocate saying 'no' to sex. Instead, we must continue our work in and outside classrooms to change the social and economic conditions that keep women and men from maximizing their potential as fully human, sexual beings."

(Trudell, 1992)

Introduction

Given the quotes above, perhaps William Yarber (1994) is stating the obvious when he writes that

The ideological conflict surrounding the question of adolescent's sexuality affects the content of sexuality education. Basically, those who believe adolescents are sexual beings advance a comprehensive approach, while those who deny adolescent sexuality want total abstinence to be promoted by education. (p. 10)

In other words, those with a Restrictive sexual ideology want sexuality education in the schools to focus exclusively on persuading children and adolescents to refrain from any type of sexual activity until marriage. Those with a Permissive sexual ideology favour what is commonly referred to as comprehensive sexuality education. Yarber (1994) describes the comprehensive approach as follows.

An important and typical tenet of this approach is that sexuality education should prepare adolescents for the healthy expression of their sexuality instead of focusing only on the prevention of negative consequences. The comprehensive approach not only deals with traditional areas such as reproductive biology and puberty, dating, marriage and STD, but also covers many topics historically considered inappropriate, such as sexual pleasure, noncoital sexual expression, sexuality and society, and homosexuality. This approach affirms the positiveness of sexuality while striving to prevent inappropriate sexual sharing and unprotected coitus. (Yarber, 1994, p. 13)

Those who favour comprehensive sexuality education in the schools are said to endorse sexual permissiveness and those who favour an abstinence-only approach to sexuality education are said to be sexual conservatives. As I will try to show in this chapter, it is accurate to say that much, if not most, of the sexuality education occurring in North American public schools is informed primarily by sexual ideology. In many cases, sexual ideology becomes *the* philosophy of education guiding the curriculum. In other words, many public school sexuality education programs are based on some fundamental premises about the nature of human sexuality and how it should be appropriately expressed. So, for example, how a sexuality education program addresses an issue like teenage pregnancy prevention is often determined by a particular ideological perspective on adolescent sexuality.

Cannaught Marshner, a leading New Right spokeswoman, has summarized well the divide between the pro-family movement and others on the matter of teenage pregnancy: "They (liberals) begin with the premise that teenagers should not have babies. We begin with the premise that single teenagers should not have sex." (Joffe, 1993, p. 287)

This divide is clearly an ideological one: Marshner is not referring here to what constitutes the most effective practical strategy for helping teenagers avoid unwanted pregnancies, but is stating a difference in moral perspective. She is articulating the moral premise of Restrictive sexual ideology which argues that teenagers should not have sex and contrasting it with the Permissive moral premise that teenagers should, and inevitably will, choose for themselves how best to prevent pregnancy.

The degree to which the Restrictive and Permissive sexual ideologies have influenced sexuality education in the schools has varied across time and place. As I will show, in some cases, contemporary public school sexuality education is overwhelmingly dominated by a particular sexual ideology. In other cases it is a melange of conflicting ideological influences. In still others, because of the ideological conflict surrounding sexuality, educational programs are, due to political expediency, lacking in substance. Examining sexuality education in terms of the extent to which it is guided by sexual ideology raises profound questions about the degree to which sexuality education functions as a form of ideological indoctrination rather than as space for students to explore and critically deliberate between different ways of thinking about sexuality.

The Influence of Restrictive Sexual Ideology on Sexuality Education

Throughout most of Western history, various forms of Restrictive sexual ideology have played a hegemonic role in guiding the sexual norms, ethics, and social policies of our culture. As a result, we can expect that, historically, the sexuality education of youth would follow the dictates of restrictive sexual ideology. According to Money (1985), we have been living, for most of our history, under an "official policy of antisexual prudery" that "distorts all public education texts for juveniles on sex education and family life" (p. 118). Consequently, "During the last 100 years...in the United States sex education materials for young people have emphasized fearful and dangerous aspects of sexuality (e.g., disease, pregnancy, behavioral abberations)" (Frayser, 1994, p. 210). In sum, just as it has traditionally guided society in general, Restrictive sexual ideology has until recently also determined to a large extent whether sexuality education would be offered in the schools and what its form and content would be if it did occur.

In recent decades, the proponents of Restrictive sexual ideology have changed their perspective toward sexuality education in the schools. Prior to the 1980s, the primary thrust of the Restrictive ideological approach to sexuality education was simply that it did not belong in the schools. "Their strategy has been to avoid the topic altogether if possible or call for parents as the only proper purveyors of sexual information" (Pollis, 1983, p. 288). At the heart of the Restrictive ideological opposition to sexuality education was the firm belief that children and adolescents had little or no need for information about human sexuality. Knowledge of sexuality was only needed as an individual prepared to enter marriage. As recently as 1987, Tim Lahaye (1987), the president of an organization called Family Life Services argued that

> Having lectured hundreds of times on the subject and having written a best-selling book on sexual adjustment in marriage, I believe we can teach most people all the basic ingredients in two or three hours just prior to marriage. (p. 57)

Phyllis Schlafly (cited in SIECUS, 1993), president of the Eagle Forum, suggests that as far as teenagers are concerned, "The facts of life can be told in fifteen minutes" (p. 17) and that teens should be told to "keep your hands out of what's inside your swimsuit—that takes care of most girls and boys" (Schlafly cited in Haffner & De Mauro, 1991, p. 19). The Restrictive ideological conceptualization of sexuality argued that a well-adjusted individual would wait for marriage to engage in sexual activity. It followed that supplying youth with sexual information was simply unnecessary. Presumably, keeping sexual information from youth would, working in conjunction with restrictive social norms upholding the virtue of premarital virginity, keep children and adolescents sexually innocent.

Furthermore, according to the Restrictive anti-sexuality education perspective, instruction in human sexuality was not only unnecessary, it was extremely dangerous. Sexuality education led to a preoccupation with sex which in turn inevitably led to promiscuity. According to psychiatrist Melvin Anchell (1987),

> Today's K through 12 sex education programs lead young people into becoming conscienceless, polymorphous sexual robots capable of en-

gaging in any kind of sex act with indifference and without guilt. (p. 52)

Many of those people who have actively opposed sexuality education in the schools did so because they "were convinced that young people who were informed about sexuality will promiscuously indulge in premarital sexual intercourse and become pregnant" (Bruess & Greenberg, 1994, p. 61).

However, from the Restrictive ideological perspective, the greatest problem with sexuality education in the schools was that it was likely to focus, in part, on the concept of decision-making, encouraging students to make at least semi-autonomous choices about their sexual behaviour. In school-based sexuality education, "Refusing sex, no less than having sex, becomes a matter of following individual dictates rather than following socially instituted and culturally enforced norms" (Dafoe-Whithead, 1994, p. 80). This violates the Restrictive ideological principle that an individual's decisions about sexual behaviour are to be derived from an external authority which prescribes pre-set standards of sexual conduct. In effect, from this view, individuals—least of all children and adolescents—should not make sexual decisions based on personal deliberation per se except to endorse the prescriptions of Restrictive sexual ideology. As long as sexuality education in the schools encouraged or focussed on decision-making it was in conflict with Restrictive sexual ideology. As I will argue later in this chapter, the focus on personal deliberation and decision-making is a primary emphasis of sexuality education informed by Permissive sexual ideology.

By the 1990s, the Restrictive ideological battle to prevent sexuality education in the schools had been lost. In response to public opinion favouring sexuality education in the schools and a growing awareness of the need to educate youth in regard to AIDS prevention, nearly all states now either mandate or recommend that sexuality and/or AIDS education be taught in the schools (Alan Guttmacher Institute, 1989; Britten, de Mauro, & Gambrell, 1992). In Canada, all the provinces and territories have school programs that include some form of sexuality education (Barrett, 1994). Having lost this battle, proponents of Restrictive sexual ideology now actively seek to have sexuality education programs that exclusively reflect their ideology implemented in the public schools. This shift in the Restrictive ideological approach to sexuality education in the schools can be summarized as follows.

> Opponents formerly argued that schools had no role in sexuality education, and that sexuality education was the sole province of parents and/or religious groups. The new strategy is for opponents of comprehensive sexuality education to define themselves as being in favour of sexuality education, so long as the curriculum exclusively emphasizes abstinence-only, or the "just say no" approach. Abstinence is defined in these curricula to mean that young people should refrain not just from sexual intercourse, but from *any* sexual activity (e.g., masturbation, breast fondling, kissing). (Scales & Roper, 1994, p. 73)

The influence of Restrictive sexual ideology on contemporary sexuality education can most readily be seen in the growing call for abstinence-only sexuality education programs in the schools and in the content of abstinence-only curricula. The arguments provided in support of abstinence-only programs, as well as the value positions promoted in abstinence-only curricula, provide an undisguised example of how these sexuality education programs are typically guided, first and foremost, by the influence of sexual ideology. The conceptual fit between Restrictive sexual ideology and abstinence-only programs such as *Sex Respect* and *Teen-Aid* is seamless.

The current abstinence-only sexuality education movement in North America can be traced to the resurgence of conservative political and social values manifested in the election of Ronald Reagan as President of the United States in 1982. Sexuality was a fundamental rallying point for the New Right. As Weeks (1986) notes, "During the 1970s and early 1980s some of the most skilful and influential developments of a politics around sexuality has come from the conservative forces, especially those grouped under the umbrella label of the New Right" (p. 89). According to Whatley and Trudell (1993), the organized campaigns to introduce *Sex Respect* and *Teen-Aid* into the schools

> must be seen in the context of a conservative resurgence over the past 15 years in government, national politics, and education. It is part of a growing backlash against gains made in the areas of civil rights, including race, gender, sexual orientation, and disability—particularly gains made by feminists. Fear-based abstinence-only curricula are part of a well-funded and well-organized political movement, the New Right, that has been increasingly able to influence public school curricula. (p. 269)

Official government support for sexuality education informed almost exclusively by Restrictive ideology was displayed with the passage of the Adolescent Family Life Act (AFLA) in 1981. The Act had "two primary purposes: the prevention of teenage pregnancy through the teaching of abstinence, and the promotion of adoption over abortion as the appropriate choice for teenagers who become pregnant" (Richards & Daley, 1994, p. 56).

Passage of the AFLA led to government funding for the development and promotion of a number of abstinence-only sexuality education curricula intended for use in the public schools, including *Sex Respect* and *Teen-Aid* (Kantor, 1994). According to former Senator Jeremiah Denton (cited in Rhode, 1993, p. 313), author of the AFLA, "The most effective oral contraceptive yet devised is the word 'no'." These programs, in accordance with Restrictive sexual ideology, promote sexual abstinence as the only viable lifestyle for unmarried persons, and reflect other Restrictive ideological positions on homosexuality, abortion, and gender. The links between abstinence-only sexuality education and right-wing or conservative ideology are well known (Eisenman, 1994; Goodson & Edmunson, 1994; Kantor, 1993; 1994; Sanderson & Wilson, 1991; Sedway, 1992; Trudell & Whatley, 1991, 1993; Yarber, 1992).

With respect to sexuality education in the schools, Restrictive sexual ideology is, for all intents and purposes, federal government policy in the United States. The welfare reform legislation signed into law by President Clinton in 1996 included a provision, not subject to public or even congressional debate, that provides $50 million in annual funding for abstinence-only sexuality education. In order to receive the federal funding, educational programs must teach "that a mutually monogamous relationship in the context of marriage is the expected standard of human sexual activity" and "that sexual activity outside of the context of marriage is likely to have harmful psychological and physical effects" (Cited in Daley, 1997, p. 3). According to a congressional document written on behalf of the authors of the legislation,

> This standard was intended to put congress on the side of social tradition...That both practices and standards in many communities across the country clash with the standard required by the law is precisely the point...the explicit goal of the abstinence-only education program is to change both behavior and community standards for the good of the country. (Cited in Daley, 1997, p. 5)

This legislation is, in no uncertain terms, a Restrictive ideological manifesto enacted as law. Prior to the 1996 abstinence-only legislation, in the United States, the *Sex Respect* curriculum had been adopted by over 1,600 school districts and other similar programs such as *Teen-Aid* are being used in many other communities (Sedway, 1992). Although *Sex Respect* has yet to gain a foothold in Canada, over 20,000 students in Saskatchewan schools are taught the *Teen-Aid* curriculum (Mitchell, 1993).

The philosophy behind these abstinence-only programs is straightforward, reflecting the moral absolutes of Restrictive sexual ideology. As a spokesperson for *Sex Respect* puts it, young people "must not only be told how to decide but also what to decide about sex. That decision should be to avoid sexual activity until marriage" (Socia, cited in Medical Institute for Sexual Health, 1993, p. 1). Furthermore,

> There is no neutral position. To simply say that it is okay to abstain conveys the idea that it is okay not to abstain. Directive abstinence teaches that the only right, good, and healthy activity is to abstain from sexual intercourse until marriage. (Socia, cited in Medical Institute for Sexual Health, 1993, p. 1)

Sex Respect was written by Colleen Kelly Mast who also authored *Love and Life: A Christian Sexual Morality Guide for Teens* (Trudell & Whatley, 1991). Thus, it is perhaps not surprising that according to Trudell and Whatley (1991), many of the recommended resources and cited sources in *Sex Respect* "are published by organizations with specific religious agendas" (p. 128). The curriculum itself is unabashed in its abstinence-only, if not anti-sex, orientation.

> The curriculum underscores the progressive *dangers* of sexual arousal in a chart that identifies the "beginning of danger" as occurring with a "prolonged kiss", with dangerous arousal increasing through "necking" and "petting" to "sexual intercourse." That chart concludes grimly with "end of relationship in its present form" (Trudell & Whatley, 1991, p. 132).

Authored by Steven Potter and Nancy Roach (1990), the *Teen-Aid* curriculum follows a similar pattern. The curriculum contains a full chapter on the advantages of abstinence but has little to say about contraception/safer sex except to point out their risks and disadvantages. Fifteen advantages of premarital abstinence are described, including "Freedom from the bother and dangers of contraceptives," "Freedom from the trauma of having to give your baby up for adoption," "Freedom to develop respect for self," "Freedom to have greater trust in marriage," and "Freedom to enjoy being a teenager" (Potter & Roach, 1990, p. 163). Meanwhile, a separate chapter, "Consequences of Adolescent Sexual Activity," begins with the message that providing teenagers with contraceptives—"birth control pills and condoms so you can have sex and not get pregnant (caught)"—is the equivalent to saying "here are some guns and getaway cars so you can steal and not get caught" (Potter & Roach, 1990, p. 163). The chapter continues with a descriptive list of the negative consequences of teen pregnancy, infection with sexually transmitted diseases, and the physical and psychological after effects of abortion.

In sum, both the *Sex Respect* and *Teen-Aid* curricula exclusively present to students a Restrictive ideological view of adolescent sexuality. Sexuality is presented in an essentially negative light and abstinence is urged as the only acceptable lifestyle for teenagers.

Although it is clear that at the curriculum content level, abstinence-only sexuality education programs vividly reflect Restrictive sexual ideology, it remains unclear as to whether these programs are philosophically grounded in accepted or popular theories of educational practice that provide a justificatory basis for exclusively encouraging abstinence. Or is it the case that with abstinence-only programs, educational practice is indelibly imprinted at its very core not so much by a philosophy of education per se but by a sexual ideology?

Within the literature advocating abstinence-only sexuality education there is little explication of the relationship between the basic tenets of the abstinence-only approach to educating youth about sexuality and the broader philosophy of education that it embraces. *Educating for Character: How Our Schools Can Teach Respect and Responsibility* by Thomas Lickona (1991), professor of Education at the State University of New York and a past president of the Association for Moral Education, provides one of the few examples of a detailed attempt to provide a justification for abstinence-only sexuality education. What is strikingly apparent from an analysis of Lickona's basic philosophical approach to educating youth about moral issues in general and his approach to educating about issues of sexual morality in particular is that the two approaches are in direct conflict. An analysis of Lickona's perspective towards these issues helps to illustrate how abstinence-only sexuality education is guided more by a sexual ideology than by a general philosophy of education. Lickona recommends Lawrence Kohlberg's well-known theory of moral development as a basis for many aspects of moral education in the schools, but recommends for sexuality education an approach to the moral aspects of sexuality that is completely contrary to Kohlberg's theory.

Taken as a whole, Kohlberg's theory of moral development and education is an inherently complex body of work (for a summary see Kohlberg, 1981; 1984). Kohlberg's approach to moral education is based on Piaget's theory of cognitive development and a moral philosophy that focusses on the principle of justice. In short,

> Kohlberg combines philosophy and psychology to explain (1) what is meant by morality and (2) how one develops more adequate modes of moral reasoning. The results of his philosophical analysis and psychological research provide teachers with a powerful rationale for, and explanation of how to promote moral growth. (Reimer, Paolitto & Hersh, 1983, p. 12)

At the heart of Kohlberg's approach to moral education is the classroom discussion of moral dilemmas as a method of facilitating students' moral development. In presenting a class with moral dilemmas, the teacher gives students an opportunity to think about and discuss conflicting value positions about the moral dilemma in question.

In *Educating for Character*, Lickona (1991) endorses Kohlberg's dilemmas approach, noting that

> With this approach, a teacher encourages students to use their own moral reasoning and allows for different responses. But at the same time the teacher challenges students to examine their reasoning and that of their peers critically. (p. 245)

Lickona argues that the use of classroom dilemmas where competing points of view are debated will help students develop the skills for rational decision-making and cites research supporting the use of classroom dilemmas in facilitating moral development.

Lickona is particularly adamant in regard to the appropriateness of using the dilemma approach for controversial social issues. In a chapter titled "Teaching Controversial Issues," Lickona (1991) discusses the necessity for young people to address controversial issues as a key aspect in helping students make "reasoned judgments about the difficult moral questions of our day" (p. 269). He cites the Vietnam war as a useful example of a controversial moral issue that can be addressed in school-based moral education. By discussing issues like the Vietnam war, students are encouraged "to arrive at their own judgements by examining conflicting points of view fairly" (Lickona, 1991, p. 270). American involvement in the Vietnam war is presented as a moral dilemma in which students are asked to "Consider all points of view and identify the assumptions behind the different viewpoints and the values behind the assumptions" (Lickona, 1991, p. 270). In sum, Lickona's recommendations for integrating controversial issues in the classroom are roughly congruent with Kohlberg's cognitive developmental approach to moral education.

In a separate chapter of "Educating for Character" Lickona (1991) turns his attention to sexuality education. Although he opens the chapter by stating that "sex education must educate young people about the moral dimensions of sexual conduct" (Lickona, 1991, p. 348), his approach for teaching about controversial issues such as premarital sex is strikingly different than it is for issues like the Vietnam war, nuclear power, and medical ethics, among others. Rather than ask students to critically examine conflicting viewpoints so they can make their own informed judgements as he does for other issues, Lickona (1991) argues that when it comes to sex "The challenge now before the schools is to help young people in every way possible to make the moral decision not to get sexually involved" (p. 349).

> The school is first and foremost an *educational* institution; as such its first duty must always be to teach children the truth and good values. The truth is that sexual activity by unmarried teenagers is harmful to them and harmful to society. The morally right value is for young people to avoid such activity. (Lickona, 1991, p. 364)

In his chapter on teaching controversial issues Lickona (1991) argues that while teachers may express their own opinions about controversial issues, the classroom should not be used as means for the inculcation of their own personal opinions and beliefs. Yet, for the controversial moral issue of premarital sex, Lickona (1991) maintains that

> Schools clearly have a responsibility to their communities—as well as to the moral growth and well-being of young people—to select sex educators who do not approve of sexual involvement by their students. (p. 373)

Lickona (1991) is clear that as far as the moral aspects of sexuality are concerned, students should not critically evaluate different points of view through Kohlberg's dilemma approach, but rather "an unambiguous commitment to the value of abstinence for teenagers gives sex education the clear ethical viewpoint needed to engage, and positively influence, students' sexual moral values" (p. 355).

It seems clear that while Lickona's approach to teaching about most controversial moral issues is compatible with Kohlberg's theory of moral development and education, his approach to sexuality education is not. In one of his few statements about how his theory could be applied to sexuality education, Kohlberg (1974) suggests that moral dilemmas of a sexual nature can be "approached as other moral dilemmas are approached—that is in a developmental rather than a preaching or indoctrinative manner" (p. 111). Rather than impose specific moral viewpoints, the teacher engages the "student in a process of thinking and dialogue about a moral issue of concern, and the process allows the student to move to the next stage of development in thinking about that issue" (Kohlberg, 1974, p. 112).

What is particularly noteworthy about Lickona's position on the teaching of sexuality education is that the primary justification for his approach is a moral one: abstinence-only sexuality education instils truth and good values. (For a similar argument favouring abstinence-only sexuality education see Kilpatrick, 1993.) Whatever the merits of Lickona's moral perspective on the issue of teenage sexuality, it is striking that he has chosen indoctrination as an educational approach for this issue but favours an approach where students use their own moral reasoning for other, nonsexual, controversial issues. How can this discrepancy be explained? Lickona offers no explanation for why his approach to teaching young people about the issue of premarital sex is so radically different from his approach for teaching about other controversial moral issues. This apparent contradiction is perhaps reflective of the tendency for sexual ideology to gain ascendancy over the basic value of freedom of belief as a guiding force behind sexuality education programs in the schools. While Lickona never discloses his own view on controversial moral issues such as the Vietnam war or abortion and is content with Kohlberg's dilemma approach for addressing these issues in the classroom, he clearly holds a Restrictive sexual ideology. This is evident not only in his statements about the virtues of teenage abstinence but also in those pertaining to the "ideal of sex within marriage."

Not surprisingly, Lickona strongly endorses *Sex Respect* and *Teen-Aid* as examples of the best kind of sexuality education.

Thomas Kelly (1986) describes four approaches to discussing controversial issues in the classroom, one of which, called *exclusive partiality*, provides an apt summation of the abstinence-only approach to sexuality education.

> This position is characterized by a deliberate attempt to induce students into accepting as correct and preferable a particular position on a controversial issue through means which consciously or unconsciously preclude an adequate presentation of competing points of view. In more authoritarian forms of exclusive partiality teachers assert or assume the correctness of a particular point of view while competing perspectives are ignored, summarily dismissed, or punitively downgraded. (p. 116)

Yarber (1992), in describing those groups who most actively support abstinence-only sexuality education, suggests that they hold what cannot be mistaken for anything other than a Restrictive sexual ideology.

> These groups adhere to an absolutist or fixed worldview ideology based on biblical authority, although some individuals and groups may be more tolerant. Adherents of this perspective believe, for example, that sexuality is basically animal passion and must be controlled, that the main goal of sex is marriage and reproduction, that sex is acceptable only in heterosexual marriages, that masturbation and same-gender relationships are forbidden, and that males are the superior gender. In other words, there is only one right way for everyone. Sexuality is dominated by fear and denial, and its expression is accompanied with shame guilt, and embarrassment. (p. 327)

While it is, for all intents and purposes, eminently clear that Restrictive sexual ideology is at work in abstinence-only curriculums, its presence is also discernable in most other forms of school-based sexuality education. There can be no question that the Restrictive ideological insistence that sexuality education actively promotes sexual abstinence pervades sexuality education in the schools. National surveys of sexuality education in the United States have found that only a small minority of states provide a balanced discussion of both abstinence and safer sex practices, the former receiving far more emphasis than the latter (Alan Guttmacher Institute, 1989; Britton, de Mauro & Gambrell, 1992). In Canada, the same approach to sexuality education can be found in some provincial ministries of education curriculum policies. For example, Prince Edward Island's Family Life Education program suggests that "Central to teaching about human sexuality is the moral and social value of abstinence from sexual intercourse as an ideal practice for unmarried persons" (P.E.I. Department of Education, 1988, p. iv). In a similar vein, the AIDS education component of New Brunswick's Health and Physical Education program suggests that "Teachers have a responsibility to promote adolescent sexual abstinence as a primary means of preventing transmission of the HIV virus" (New Brunswick Department of Education, 1989, p. 1).

The province of Manitoba's Department of Education and Training's student objectives for Family Life Education illustrate the tendency toward Restrictive sexual ideology in contemporary sexuality education. While among the list of student objectives is "an appreciation of sexual abstinence as both a health and moral value among young people" and "an understanding of the risks and consequences of adolescent sexual activity" (Manitoba Education and Training, 1990, p. 6), none of the objectives refer to things such as an appreciation of the health value of consistent condom use among sexually active young people.

The Dutch sexologist Jany Rademakers (1995), in reviewing an American publication on model programs for teenage pregnancy prevention, offers the following observation on the apparent emphasis on promoting abstinence in sexuality education.

> From my (Dutch) point of view, the amount of effort aimed at either sexual abstinence or the postponement of first sexual intercourse is astounding....Instead of teaching teenagers to behave responsibly and maturely in this respect, for example, by encouraging them to choose their own time, place, and conditions to have intercourse, they are more or less explicitly told that having intercourse is wrong for teenagers. This moralistic message is often defended with a practical argument: the logical fact that less teenagers having intercourse results in less teenagers at risk for unintended pregnancy. But the same applies, for example, to car accidents and no one would think about forbidding people to drive a car or postponing the age one can get a driving license. The question program designers and authors should really answer is: Would they consider it bad for teenagers to have sexual intercourse when they would protect themselves effectively against pregnancy and AIDS and sexually transmitted diseases (STD)? When they answer this question affirmatively, their restrictive attitude

toward teenage sexuality becomes evident, whereas all others can start aiming their activities at the real problem: unsafe sexual behavior. (pp. 359-360)

It is clear that, if they were candid about it, many of those who profess a Restrictive ideological approach to sexuality education would answer in the affirmative to Rademaker's query.

The Influence of Permissive Sexual Ideology on Sexuality Education

It is difficult to discern the specific influences of Permissive sexual ideology on contemporary sexuality education in the schools. Because Permissive sexual ideology emerged out of a culture in which Restrictive sexual ideology was, until relatively recently, largely hegemonic, the Permissive influence on sexuality education has been somewhat diffuse. Sexuality education has always been controversial and when confronted with opposing views "government reaction has occurred primarily in the direction of fundamentalism" (Neutens, 1992, p. 72). In other words, because sexuality education programs informed by Permissive sexual ideology take place within a larger culture that is heavily influenced by Restrictive sexual ideology, few of these programs have completely escaped the cultural weight of Restrictive ideology. For example, whereas sexuality education based on Restrictive sexual ideology exclusively promotes abstinence, programs informed by Permissive sexual ideology frequently bend to Restrictive sexual ideology by complementing discussions of safer-sex not just with a discussion of abstinence but with the recommendation that abstinence is the "most effective" or "best way" to prevent unwanted pregnancy and STDs (e.g., see American School Health Association, 1991, p. 111; Frost & Darroch Forrest, 1995, p. 190; Yarber, 1993, p. 22).[1] Indeed, the Restrictive ideological belief that educators should be in the business of promoting sexual abstinence among teenagers has become so accepted that even educators who would be considered Permissive in their approach to sexuality education often actively lobby adolescents to be abstinent. For example, as Joffe (1993) explains

it is in fact not only pro-family adherents who believe in sexual abstinence for teenagers. Many, if not most, "liberals" who work directly in the field of pregnancy prevention also deeply believe in the

desirability of the choice of abstinence for teenagers, and they actively
promote this option. (p. 287)

Although some form of Restrictive sexual ideology is present in most, if
not all, sexuality education programs in the schools, the mere existence of
school-based sexuality education is testimony to the powerful influence of
Permissive sexual ideology. In addition, many of the precepts of Permissive
sexual ideology have become the guiding principles of many sexuality
education programs. Indeed, conservative critics have pointed to the
influence of Permissive sexual ideology as a justification for condemning
current forms of sexuality education in the schools. For example, according
to Barbara Dafoe Whitehead (1994),

> The unifying core of comprehensive sex education is not intellectual
> but ideological. Its mission is to defend and extend the freedoms of
> the sexual revolution, and its architects are called forth from a variety
> of pursuits to advance this cause. (p. 70)

Whereas I have earlier suggested that the unifying core of abstinence-only
sexuality education is Restrictive sexual ideology, Dafoe Whitehead is
making a similar argument about the relationship between Permissive sexual
ideology and comprehensive sexuality education. An analysis of the evolution of contemporary sexuality education in the schools shows that this
argument is not without foundation.

Of the architects of modern sexuality education, Mary Calderone was
perhaps the most influential. A medical doctor by profession and former
Medical Director of the Planned Parenthood Federation of America, Calderone co-founded the Sex Information and Education Council of the
United States (SIECUS) in 1964. She served as the executive director of
SIECUS for more than five years and remained a key SIECUS spokesperson
for many years afterward. Through the 1960s and 1970s, Calderone worked
diligently to further the cause of sexuality education. Szasz (1982) refers to
her as "the founding mother of modern sex education" (p. 124). While
many, if not most people, would applaud Calderone's efforts to see that
young people have the opportunity to learn about human sexuality, her
critics are quick to point out that her views on the proper nature of sexuality
education were liberal and permissive (e.g., Reisman & Eichel, 1990; Szasz,
1982). On one level, Calderone was seen as liberal and permissive because
she advocated "a good, basic, window-opening course of education for

sexuality" (Calderone cited in Mass, 1990, p. 68), a view that few Restrictive ideologues shared during the 1960s and 1970s.

It is apparent that at the time Calderone was advocating the right of people to receive sexuality education, she believed, with some justification, that the primary obstacle to providing such education was the religiously inspired taboos surrounding sexuality. These taboos kept basic sexual information out of the reach of most people. Her solution was to separate sexuality from religion and its moral dictates and link it instead with the concept of health. When asked in an interview if this was her purpose, Calderone responded:

> Yes, and that turned out to be wise because it took sex out of the realm of morals. Fundamentally, sex has always been preempted by the religions and everybody kept hands off. By putting it into the area of health, where it scientifically belongs, by recognizing its role in physical, mental, and social well-being, we immediately freed it for objective, less emotional study and consideration. (cited in Szasz, 1982, p. 122)

Calderone's statement that linking sex with health "took sex out of the realm of morals" reflects the common, but faulty, assumption that sexual morality is equivalent to religious morality. This statement is deceptive because Calderone did not take a moral-free approach to her philosophy of sexuality education. In fact, she invoked a basic moral principle in saying that "sexual self determination is clearly what sex education is all about" (Calderone, cited in Szasz, 1982, p. 123). In chronicling the sexuality education controversy in the United States during the 1960s, Breasted (1970), although highly critical of the Right-wing opponents of sexuality education, discerned in Calderone's writing and speeches "a willingness to present the truth selectively to youngsters. Instead of a propaganda by polemics, she was in favor of filtering material to them that supported her views on morality" (p. 238). In terms of the morality of premarital sexual intercourse, it is clear that while Calderone had no qualms about advising teenagers of the medical and emotional risks of premarital sex, she also argued for the provision of contraceptives to young unmarried couples (Breasted, 1970, p. 237). Kobler (1972) describes Calderone's moral perspective as follows:

> As to sexual morality, Dr. Calderone is no absolutist. "Do's" and "don'ts," she believes, cannot be imposed on the young by fiat. They

simply won't accept them. In her own moral code the key words are
"exploitation" and "responsibility." Sex with no object except tran-
sient physical pleasure she scorns as the crassest exploitation of one's
partner. A moral person considers the welfare not only of the opposite
sex but also of family and society. Though Dr. Calderone feels that
the odds against a responsible, meaningful sexual relationship outside
of marriage are overwhelming, she concedes the possibility. "But
[before making any decision on the subject] young people should be
given all the information and help *to make a good decision.*" (p. 136).

Although one can discern elements of the Romanticist variant of Restrictive sexual ideology in this perspective, it is essentially permissive in nature.
The rejection of moral absolutes in favour of more pragmatic considerations
such as the welfare of others is characteristic of Permissive sexual ideology.
The notion that a morally valid sexual relationship can occur outside of
marriage is also a clear marker of Permissive sexual ideology.

The ideology behind Calderone's and SIECUS's philosophy of sexuality
is evident in SIECUS's mission statement during the 1960s, which was as
follows:

> To establish man's sexuality as a health entity: to identify the special
> characteristics that distinguish it from, yet relate it to, human repro-
> duction; to dignify it by openness of approach, study, and scientific
> research designed to lead towards its understanding and its freedom
> from exploitation; to give leadership to professionals and to society, to
> the end that human beings may be aided toward responsible use of the
> sexual faculty and toward assimilation of sex into their individual life
> patterns as a creative and re-creative force. (Breasted, 1970, pp.
> 206-207)

This mission statement is clearly not ideologically neutral. In commenting
on contemporary SIECUS positions, Ruenzel (1993) argues that

> There is in the SIECUS materials an earnestness about sexual matters
> that seems far removed from moral lassitude. It seems to me, rather,
> that SIECUS has values to which its opponents simply object. Chief
> among these values, according to the group's mission statement and
> guidelines, is the importance of conveying sexuality as "a natural and
> healthy part of life," be it heterosexual or homosexual expression. The
> goal of comprehensive sex education, a SIECUS fact sheet reads, "is
> to assist children in understanding a positive view of sexuality..." (p.
> 25)

To SIECUS' credit, it should be acknowledged that the organization's current position on sexuality education is far more ideologically inclusive and broadly-based than the views expressed by its Restrictive opponents. SIECUS is not opposed to the introduction of different ideological perspectives into the classroom. This is clearly seen in the 1991 *SIECUS Guidelines for Comprehensive Sexuality Education* which, for example, advocate the teaching of both abstinence and contraception to teenagers. Indeed, the *SIECUS Guidelines* suggest that teenagers be taught that "Most religions teach that sexual intercourse should only occur in marriage" and that "Abstinence from intercourse has benefits for teenagers" (National Guidelines Taskforce, 1991). To the extent that current SIECUS policy encourages students to contemplate both Restrictive and Permissive ideological perspectives on sexual morality and sexual health, it represents a significant departure from the tradition of overt ideological bias in American sexuality education.

Nevertheless, Calderone's approach to sexuality and sexuality education was reflective of Permissive sexual ideology in three distinct ways. First, viewed in the historical context of the 1960s, Calderone's belief in the virtues of sexuality education in the schools, providing sexual information to young people, was characteristic of Permissive sexual ideology. During this period, those with a Restrictive sexual ideology generally opposed the idea of sexuality education in the schools. Secondly, the reliance on science, as opposed to religion, as the explanatory framework that would deliver the goods on what constitutes responsible sexuality reflects the philosophy of Naturalism which informs much of Permissive sexual ideology. Thirdly, the sexual ethics that Calderone proposed as a framework for sexuality education was, at the very least, sympathetic to Permissive sexual ideology.

The adoption of a Naturalist conceptualization of human sexuality is perhaps the most easily discernable influence that Permissive sexual ideology has had on contemporary sexuality education programs in the schools. As I noted in Chapter Two, Naturalists conceptualize the nature of human sexuality, not from the standpoint of spirituality as Jehovanists do, but rather from the standpoint of science and nature. Sexuality, from the Naturalist point of view, is simply one of many more or less "natural" parts of life. This view is reflected in Mauro's (1990) survey of sexuality education programs of the public schools which found that "two thirds of the curricula affirm that sexuality is a natural part of life" (p. 7).[2]

It is clear that the most common theme in modern sexuality education in the schools is a focus on the biology of reproduction and STDs. In fact, it is often the case that sexuality education consists of little else aside from biology. While few would disagree with the idea that sexuality education should include biological information, programs that rely exclusively on the science of biology as an explanatory framework for learning about human sexuality should not be seen as completely neutral in their approach. As Whatley (1987) points out in her analysis of contemporary sexuality education, "The scientific approach to sexuality can easily lead to a view in which the 'laws of nature' neatly coincide with a political agenda" (p. 29).[3]

Although biologically-based sexuality education is frequently viewed as ideologically innocuous, particularly by its proponents, it is clearly compatible with Naturalist sexual ideology. As Davis (1983) argues, "Although Naturalists believe that their sex education courses teach children about sex in an unbiased way, they actually proselytize Naturalist metaphysics by depicting a cosmos in which sex is merely a neutral, natural, harmless activity like any other" (p. 243). While neither the proponents of Restrictive sexual ideology nor those of Permissive sexual ideology are content with the reduction of sexuality education to the provision of strictly biological information related to reproduction and STDs, such education is more likely to conform to Permissive sexual ideology in that it fails to prescribe strict limits on sexual behaviour.

The adoption of values clarification as a method of exploring ethical issues related to sexuality is perhaps the most potent example of the influence of Permissive sexual ideology on the history of modern sexuality education. During the 1960s and 1970s, the forces of Permissive sexual ideology began to have some success in introducing sexuality education into the public school classroom. However, in attempting to articulate the moral context in which sexuality education would take place, these educators were caught in a catch-22. On one hand, the advocates of sexuality education were keenly aware that their programs needed to avoid any hint of moral indoctrination. Substantiated accusations that sexuality education was enforcing a particular set of moral, most likely Permissive, prescriptions would be catastrophic to the cause of sexuality education. This led to the popularization of the idea of a "value-free" or "value neutral" sexuality education. The idea of a value-free sexuality education was appealing because it would achieve the dual purpose of freeing programs from the rigid morality of Restrictive sexual ideology and of removing the spectre of indoctrination. As Andrew Greely (1988) writes, "In the minds of most people, to have values about sex means to be saddled with a heavy baggage of moral prohibitions" (p. xiv). Since "a heavy baggage of moral prohibitions" did not correspond to Permissive sexual ideology, the proponents of sexuality education often portrayed themselves as taking a value-free approach. Morris (1994) describes the appeal of a value-free approach to sexuality education.

> Some social scientists in this period argued that sexuality education should remain value-free. Louis Karmel (1970), for example, argued that sexuality education should be limited to "sex information." This information should impart "biological and mechanistic data without prescribing how these impulses should not be channelled" (p. 95). Karmel saw the teaching of values-related areas as inappropriate for public schools given the growing pluralism of American society and given the lack of certainty about value issues. (pp. 7-8)

With the 1966 publication of *Values and Teaching* by Raths, Harmin, and Simon the values clarification movement began to gain currency. The book has been a standard text for training teachers to teach moral education in the classroom (Carter, 1984, p. 49). Values clarification became a popular model of moral education during the 1970s. Its rise to prominence can be attributed to the growing recognition in educational circles of the need to conceptualize moral education in a way that accommodated the growing moral pluralism of American society. This pluralism, it is argued, leads to "value confusion."

> Values clarification advocates point out that within "value-rich" areas such as politics, religion, friendship, love, sex, race, and money, decision making is subject to many influences. Students are exposed to parental, peer, school, and religious influences, which often contradict one another. The effects of such variables as working parents, broken homes, television, big schools, different teachers, a variety of friends, and travel often result in value confusion. (Hersh, Miller, & Fielding, 1980, p. 74)

Values clarification would help young people overcome their value confusion.

According to the principle architects of this theory, many of the problems experienced by young people "are profitably seen as caused by a lack of values" (Raths, Harmin, & Simon, 1978, p. 10). Those who lack values tend, it is claimed, to be flighty, apathetic, uncertain, inconsistent, drifting, overconforming, and overdissenting. Those, however, who develop a clear sense of what their values are in the relationship between themselves and society will be more likely to exhibit qualities of being positive, purposeful, enthusiastic, proud and consistent. This approach is not necessarily value free, but rather attempts to remain value neutral by limiting itself to helping students clarify what their values are.

The goal of values clarification is to help students develop the desired qualities by participating in class exercises involving a seven-step valuing process. Once students are accustomed to addressing value related issues through reference to the seven-step process they will exhibit the desired qualities typical of those who are able to have a clear sense of their own values. The seven steps of values clarification are: choosing freely; choosing from alternatives; choosing after consideration of the consequences; prizing and cherishing; affirming; acting upon choices; and repeating (Raths, Harmin, & Simon, 1978).

Values clarification has become a common way of addressing value-related issues in sexuality education. It is a frequently proposed strategy within the sexuality education literature (e.g., Bruess & Greenberg, 1994; Lohrman, 1987; Morrison & Price, 1974; Vincent & Pfefferkarn, 1994). In Canada, surveys of teachers (Lawlor & Purcell, 1988) and curriculum guidelines (Ajzenstat & Gentles, 1988) suggest that values clarification is the preferred approach. According to Morris (1994) "This is by far the most popular position on values in sexuality education" (p. 11).

Morris (1994) summarizes the rationale for the integration of values clarification into sex education.

> Although proponents of values clarification reject the idea that sexuality education should be value-*free*, they do argue that teachers should remain value-*neutral*. They argue that teachers should be non-judgemental and should convey to students that there are no right or wrong answers. Since values are viewed as personal and subjective, the teachers role is to ex-pose but not im-pose values. Sexuality education, the argument goes, ought to encourage decision-making by helping students *clarify* their *own* values (p. 11).

However, as Morris (1994) notes, even this type of presumably value-neutral sexuality education was vigorously denounced by Right wing groups who maintained that any type of sexuality education in the schools "would lead to moral perversion and the disintegration of the family" (p. 8).

In the end, the value-free approach was unworkable, leading to a "catch-22" in that although sexuality educators had now side-stepped the potential accusation of moral indoctrination, they were now susceptible to accusations of an even more heinous crime: implying, albeit perhaps unintentionally, that sexuality itself need not be subjected to rigorous moral analysis. This was highly problematic since most people will agree, no matter their ideology, that sexuality and morality are inextricably linked. In sum, sexuality educators had a dilemma on their hands in that they had a difficult time articulating a way in which they could refrain from indoctrination on one hand, and avoid being highly relativistic on the other.

As we saw in Chapter Two, Permissive sexual ideology is not without moral substance. Although its opponents have sometimes tried to portray the sexual ethics of Permissive sexual ideology as being extremely relativistic, if not entirely subjective, it is more likely that most people who hold a Permissive sexual ideology champion secular moral principles such as mutual consent, reciprocity, and fairness as the basis for sexual ethics. Nearly all of those with a Permissive sexual ideology will agree with the idea that it is an "undeniable fact that a considerable part of managing sexuality also involves managing social relationships" (Gagnon & Simon, 1973, p. 123) and that the way one's actions in a particular situation affect the welfare of others is a major component of morality (Rest, 1984). Thus from this perspective, if sexuality is viewed in its relational context, it becomes an important topic for critical discourse from the standpoint of social morality (Darling & Mabe, 1989). However, driven by the imperative to avoid community controversy and charges of indoctrination, the advocates of sexuality education, most of whom held a Permissive sexual ideology, in many respects betrayed their ideology's moral perspective by embracing the openly relativistic values clarification approach as their way of integrating values into sexuality education.

It is, perhaps, self-evident that when Restrictive ideologues assert that public schools must insist that their students adopt an abstinence-only standard of conduct, they are promoting indoctrination: telling students what to think rather than exploring different ways of thinking. It is, perhaps, less self-evident, but often no less true, that Permissive ideologues, through the promotion of values clarification in sexuality education, are guilty of a similar offense. But doesn't values clarification encourage and respect students freedom of belief? The answer is yes, but only within the confines of Permissive sexual ideology. Among the fundamental steps of the valuing process in values clarification is the task of choosing between alternatives. Making such choices is fully consistent with the ethics of Permissive sexual ideology. They are, in fact, an exercise in decision-making within the Permissive ideological framework of sexual ethics. The philosophical adequacy of these exercises may even be enhanced, to become more reflective of the essence of Permissive sexual ideology, with the introduction of substantive moral criteria such as considerations of honesty, equality, fairness, etc. What needs to be made very clear, however, is that while choosing among alternatives is a staple of Permissive sexual ideology, it is antithethical to Restrictive sexual ideology. From a Restrictive ideological perspective, addressing a question like "Should I have premarital sex?" does not involve choosing between the alternatives of becoming sexually active or remaining abstinent until marriage: one follows the moral absolute that sex before marriage is immoral. Values clarification exercises rarely ask students to clarify their religious beliefs or basic philosophy of life. Rather, they typically present a concrete dilemma to be solved through the process of choosing among alternative solutions to a specific situation. This is at odds with the core principles of Restrictive sexual ideology. For example, adhering to natural law theory does not mean choosing among alternatives, it means learning and applying moral absolutes.

Ajzenstat and Gentiles (1988) note that the values clarification approach is directly contrary to the sexual ethics espoused by most religious and ethical traditions which rely on, in their words, "objective standards" for decision-making. It may be inferred that what the authors mean by "objective standards" is the moral absolutes of Restrictive sexual ideology.[4]

> We would add that virtually any of the world's religions or ethical traditions could furnish the framework of an "objective standards" based sex education program. Globally speaking, it is hard to think of an ethical/religious tradition, apart from Western liberal utilitarianism, that would sanction a "personal values" approach.(Ajzenstat & Gentiles, 1988, p. 61)

The important issue here is that it would appear that many sexuality education programs do not offer students an impartial opportunity to differentiate and ultimately choose between the "objective standards" that are the moral absolutes of Restrictive sexual ideology and the "liberal utilitarianism" of Permissive sexual ideology. Rather, the values clarification, used by so many sexuality education programs, seems to validate Permissive sexual ethics as a preferred form of moral judgement.

Values in Sexuality: A New Approach to Sex Education written in 1974 by Morrison and Price contains a large number of values clarification exercises designed to be used in the sexuality education classroom. Although the authors contend that "the approach in this book precludes endorsement or condemnation of any particular point of view with regard to sexual codes" (Morrison & Price, 1974, p. 11), many of the values clarification exercises contained in the book are conducive only to the parameters of Permissive sexual ideology. For example, the first exercise in the values clarification section of the book asks students to answer the following multiple choice question, "For me, it is most important that a sexual experience: a. Be fun and pleasurable. b. Increase the possibility of honesty and openness. c. Enhance self-respect" (Morrison & Price, 1974, p. 97). All of these choices are reasonable within a Permissive ideological perspective. However, none of the three choices conforms, in any direct way, with the dictates of Restrictive sexual ideology. If the list of choices had included "Has the potential to result in procreation within a marital relationship" or "Contributes to the loving bond of a mature marital relationship" then one could at least argue that the possibility of choosing an option reflective of Restrictive sexual ideology was possible within the boundaries of the exercise. Other exercises follow the same pattern. For example, students are asked to complete the following item: "In a sexual relationship, I would prefer that: a. Sex be more meaningful to me than to the other person. b. Sex be more meaningful to the other person than me. c. Sex be meaningful to neither one of us" (p. 99). None of these possible answers are amenable to Restrictive sexual ideology.

In sum, values clarification reflects Permissive sexual ideology in two distinct ways. First, students are encouraged to repeatedly make deliberated choices about specific sexual issues. They are not being asked to clarify their ideological perspective as a precursor to discussing these issues, but rather are being sent the explicit message that choosing among alternatives is the preferred method for doing sexual ethics. This reflects Permissive sexual ideology, but is directly contrary to Restrictive sexual ideology. Secondly, as the two examples given above show, the alternative choices provided in most exercises of this kind exclusively fit Permissive sexual ideology.[5] Restrictive ideologues may have a point when they accuse the proponents of values clarification in sexuality education of attempting to rig the proceedings in favour of Permissive sexual ideology. It might even be argued that the integration of values clarification into sexuality education represents a covert attempt to introduce an exclusive partiality representing Permissive sexual ideology. As Kelly (1986) notes,

> Whether the advocacy and dismissal is done passionately or matter of factly, haphazardly or more systematically, the sum effect is a one-sided presentation where challenge to the preferred point of view is discouraged or precluded. In more subtle forms of partiality, the teacher may give the appearance of permitting genuine dialogue and dissent yet nevertheless attempt to stack the deck. (p. 116)

In other words, while values clarification is, at first glance, impartial with regards to divergent sexual ideologies, it is fully compatible only with Permissive sexual ideology.

The Bare-Bones Approach to Sexuality Education in the Schools

There is another form of sexuality education in the schools which is far more prevalent than those which are exclusively partial to either Restrictive or Permissive sexual ideology. This is not a form of sexuality education that impartially allows students to explore, critically evaluate, and affirm or reject various sexual ideologies. Nor is it a form of sexuality education that encourages students to clarify their own ideological perspectives and debate their implications for self and society. Nor does this form of education provide students with a broad base of information which they need to protect their health. This most prevalent form of sexuality education does none of these things. It is what I call the *bare-bones* approach to sexuality education and it occurs precisely because of our society's ideological conflict around sexuality.

Because there is a pervasive conflict of sexual ideologies in Western society, it is often the case that sexuality educators go to extraordinary lengths to avoid offending the proponents of both Restrictive and Permissive sexual ideology. Sexuality educators have, as Whatley (1992) writes, "picked up the strong message that it is dangerous to teach about sexuality and that every care must be taken to avoid attracting notice or stirring up controversy" (p. 78). Many educators, as we have seen, respond to the threat of controversy by claiming a nonpartisan or neutral status for their sexuality education as they relate to different ideological perspectives on sexuality. However, in most cases, the chosen strategy to accomplish this feat is not to teach in a way that is inclusive of different ideological perspectives for this itself would cause controversy. Rather, the chosen strategy is to omit from the program any topic that is the subject of ideological dispute. As Neutens (1994) suggests,

> While the conservative and liberal camps fight over "what's right" and "what's wrong," those in the middle are left in a moral smog that compounds an already difficult decision-making process. As a result of the moral smog, well-founded program objectives may be diluted or distorted at the local level. (p. 30)

Kelly (1986) describes this approach to education as a position of *exclusive neutrality*. It is the idea that "teachers should not introduce into the curriculum any topics which are controversial in the broader community" (p. 114). Such exclusion, it is argued, "allegedly preserves the nonpartisan or neutral status of the school" (Ibid.).

There is no question that what passes for sexuality education in the schools most often consists of little more than the most cursory provision of knowledge about human sexuality. As Haffner (1992) puts it, "Although most young people receive some type of sexuality education before they graduate from high school, what is labelled sexuality or family life education is often little more than teaching about biology, reproduction, and virology" (p. vii). A number of surveys of the content of sexuality education programs in the United States clearly indicate that most programs are characterized by the omission of fundamental aspects of human sexuality (Britton, Mauro, & Gambril, 1992; Calamidas, 1990; Forrest & Silverman, 1989; Holtzman & Greene, 1992; Mauro, 1990). For example, one review of state sexuality and AIDS education curricula in the United States found that,

> few provide information on the historical and cultural aspects of human sexuality, sexual values, attitudes, beliefs, sexual activities and functioning. Fewer than one in ten include any information on sexual behaviors. Almost half of the curricula limited information about family planning. In fact, fewer than one in six of the state curricula provide young people with a comprehensive base of information and education. (Mauro, 1990, p. 7)

Because sexuality is so controversial, for school administrators and educators, the safest possible position to take is that of exclusive neutrality: the omission from sexuality education of any substantive base of critical thought and knowledge.

Conclusion

Based on a series of interviews with the proponents of both abstinence-only and comprehensive sexuality education, Nelson (1996) articulates the ideological context and scope of the battle over sexuality education in the schools.

> My interviews with advocates of comprehensive sexuality education show a deep concern that abstinence-only education is part of a crusade to transform contemporary American society into an authoritarian theocracy.
>
> Similarly, my interviews with the proponents of abstinence-only education suggest that their opposition is based upon a belief that comprehensive sexuality education is a component in "relativist" ideology where students will learn to choose their own sexual values.
>
> The work of both groups stems not only from their desire to promote specific sexual ideologies and societal visions but also from their perception that the opposition represents a crucial component in a hostile and encroaching political movement.
>
> As such, the debated curricula are manifest symbols in a much larger cultural struggle over which of the two group's visions of morality, family, and gender will predominate. (p. 16)

In this chapter, I have tried to demonstrate how the ideological underpinnings of the Restrictive and Permissive sexual ideologies have influenced the form and content of sexuality education in the schools. I have described three tendencies that shape sexuality education. The first two—sexuality education informed by Restrictive and Permissive sexual ideology—represent exclusive partiality: the explicit or implicit imposition of a particular sexual ideology. The third and most prevalent tendency is for sexuality education to take a position of exclusive neutrality: the omission of any subject matter which might be deemed to be controversial. Which, if any, of these three forms of sexuality education is preferable? Should it be Restrictive or Permissive sexual ideology that informs public policy related to sexuality, including sexuality education in the schools?

Notes

1. The assertion that "abstinence is the best way to prevent pregnancy and STDs" appears to be a taken-for-granted assumption within the public and professional discourse on adolescent sexuality and sexuality education. However, abstinence is only "the best way" if an individual or couple is, of their own accord, willing to forsake the potential benefits of sexual activity. The statement seems to assume that all rational adolescents would choose abstinence—an issue that certainly could be debated. Do all adolescents who choose to become sexually active do so irrationally? An analogous statement that frequently appears in sexuality education curricula is that "abstinence is the only 100% effective means of pregnancy and STD prevention." However, this statement is only true in-so-far as the individual who chooses abstinence is able to abide by that choice consistently. Many people who make vows of abstinence are unable to keep them. History certainly shows us that if abstinence is to be considered a birth-control method, it is far less than 100% effective. Indeed, a study of American contraceptive practices found that of people who report that they use abstinence as their method of contraception, 26% become pregnant each year (Jones & Forrest, 1992). Both of these statements are perhaps indicative of how certain Restrictive ideological assumptions are so deeply ingrained in our culture that they are rarely questioned.

2. That this tendency to affirm the Permissive ideological notion that sexuality is a *natural* part of life appears to coexist with Restrictive ideological notions, such as the abstinence-only imperative, suggests that the content of contemporary sexuality education in the schools is influenced by a melange of often contradictory ideological influences. One can imagine that some students may have difficulty grasping the concept that although sexuality is a natural part of their lives, they must resist their inclinations for sexual expression.

3. It is not only those with a Restrictive sexual ideology who oppose a strictly biological approach to sexuality education. For example, both Sears (1992) and Whatley (1987) are concerned that this type of sexuality education de-emphasizes the pleasurable aspects of sexuality and may reinforce prevailing gender stereotypes by, perhaps inadvertently, promoting biological determinism.

4. Ajzenstat and Gentiles (1988, p. 45) cite programs that are "deeply rooted in Judeo-Christian values" or that encourage students to behave in ways that "will be in keeping with their duties to God, themselves, and society" as examples of sexuality education that promotes "objective standards."

5. It should be acknowledged that some of the exercises provided by Morrison and Price do allow for the expression of views amenable to Restrictive sexual ideology. For example, one exercise asks students to consider a number of specific sexual activities with the aim of having individual students clarify

whether the activity is "Acceptable to me, Does not matter to me," or is "Unacceptable to me." Indeed, such an exercise may be quite useful in helping students clarify their ideological position.

CHAPTER FOUR

Discovering the Truth About Sexuality

■··■—■—··■—■——··■—·——··—··■—··——··—■—··

> There is no easy way to decide who is right because, like scientific
> paradigms, each interpretive sexual scheme determines the very facts
> by which it justifies itself.
>
> (Davis, 1983)
>
> In observing the mote in our opponent's eye we may have become blind
> to the beam in our own.
>
> (Smart, 1995)

Introduction

The opinion that the sexual norms, values, and social policies related
to sexuality in contemporary Western culture are in a state of good repair
is very seldom heard. Rather, we are constantly inundated with reports of
how sexuality manifests itself in psychopathology, and ruptures relationships, is a weapon of power, exploitation, and injustice, and leads to disease,
death, and social and moral decay. Neither those with a Restrictive nor
those with a Permissive ideological bent appear to be altogether happy with
the sexual state of the union. It appears that most of us can agree,
irrespective of our ideology, that the Western sexual landscape is in need of
some reform.

Because this disapproval of the sexual status quo comes from all sides
of the ideological spectrum, finding a consensus on how we, as a society, can
reach for constructive change has unfortunately eluded us. The result is
personal, social, and public policy paralysis. We continue to immerse
ourselves in a never ending debate over which sexual ideology is right and
good. At best, we might hope to engage in a comparative, presumably
objective, critical assessment of the Restrictive and Permissive sexual ideologies in order to draw some conclusion about which ideology, or some

form of it, seems most reasonable in the sense that it corresponds to the essential and true nature of human sexuality and reflects sound moral reasoning. By drawing a conclusion of this kind, we might want to create and implement social policies, including those involving sexuality education in the schools, that are based on the superior ideology, perhaps intending to impose them on the adherents of the inferior ideology. But is it possible to arrive at a definitive and objective conclusion about the true nature and purpose of human sexuality? The nature of ideology combined with the indisputable fact of an intransigent pluralism related to sexual morality in our culture should teach us that this zero-sum game contest between sexual ideologies is both delusionary and unwinnable. Furthermore, as I shall discuss in subsequent chapters, definitively declaring, if it were possible, a final winner in the moral validity contest between Restrictive and Permissive sexual ideology would be profoundly at odds with the ideals of a democratic culture.

In this chapter I will argue that one cannot conclusively demonstrate the superiority of a particular sexual ideology in either a scientific or philosophical sense. This being the case, I will propose in Chapter Five that our collective approach, as a society, to issues of sexual morality ought to be based not on a particular sexual ideology as the public ethos, but on a larger democratic perspective that acknowledges ideological diversity and the right of individuals and groups to hold, and live by, different sexual ideologies. In Chapters Six and Seven, I will explore the implications of this democratic perspective for sexuality education.

Can We Discover the Truth About Sexuality?

Can we as a society arrive at a truth about sexuality that is independent of ideology? This question can be addressed in a number of ways but all of them raise doubts about the likelihood of finding universal non-ideological truths about the nature of human sexuality and sexual ethics. In general, part of the problem in finding *the truth* about sexuality is that it is very difficult to come at these issues in a completely detached way. When we discover something about the sexual we discover something about ourselves both individually and as a society. At the personal level, our values may be supported or refuted, our desires and emotional responses normalized or pathologized, our identity affirmed or questioned. At the societal level, our inquiries into the nature of sexuality can dramatically shape our perceptions of appropriate social policy regarding fundamental aspects of the social order. In sum, there is much at stake when we seek the truth about sexuality. Since we are all sexual beings to some extent, with identities, attitudes, and values, it is not hard to see why bringing an impartial eye to finding an ideology-free truth about sexuality is a highly problematic project. Although this observation seems self evident as a matter of simple common sense, the same type of critique, focussing on the problems encountered in attempting to objectively explore human sexuality, provides solid grounds for being sceptical of the truth claims about sexuality that emerge from scientific, theological, or philosophical discourse.

Assessing the potential of the various empirical and social sciences to deliver the truth about sexuality, and to provide value-free, unbiased criteria to determine the validity of Restrictive and Permissive sexual ideologies, easily, or perhaps necessarily, slides into an interpretive evaluation of the concept of objectivity as it pertains to empirical observation and moral philosophy. While my inquiry into sexual ideology does imply a questioning of our empirical and moral objectivity in sexual matters, my focus is not on solving the philosophical puzzle of objectivity per se, but on presenting a reasonable justification for questioning a claim that either Restrictive or Permissive sexual ideology entails a reality-revealing set of indisputable facts that captures the true essence of human sexuality and its appropriate role in social life. Although one might argue that the question of sexual ideology is ultimately answered in terms of our ability to think and examine objectively, I will base my case on the assertion that sexual ideologies correspond to complex socially derived assumptions rather than on a set of value free objective facts which can be easily demonstrated.

In sum, I am taking a social constructionist approach to the analysis of sexual ideology and I hope to show that this provides a convincing case for the need not only to acknowledge ideological diversity but also to understand it in a way that allows us, no matter what our own sexual ideology is, to affirm the right of others to hold beliefs about sexuality that are contrary to our own. As I shall discuss in greater detail later in this chapter, acceptance and affirmation of diversity of sexual ideology does not deny that truth exists but only that it is contingent upon the ideological world view in which the truth is sought. The higher order question then becomes one of how we live in a society where no one truth about sexuality is likely to prevail universally.

In matters of sexuality, which are imbued with intense individual and social importance, affirming the right of others to hold beliefs about sexuality that oppose our own is exceedingly difficult. We have been reduced to accusing opposing ideologies of being wrong headed, destructive, unhealthy, morally bankrupt, and discriminatory. A social constructionist analysis of sexual ideology may provide an initial foundation for moving away from an intellectual and sociosexual framework that pushes us to wage the war of ideological superiority towards a more pluralist acceptance of diversity. This requires that we, as sexual ideologues of all stripes, begin to approach issues of sexuality and sexuality education in ways to which we, in our society, are unaccustomed. We are familiar and comfortable making the, often unconscious, assumption that *our truth* is *the truth* of the universe: the way things really are. Seeing *our truth* as a truth that corresponds not necessarily to the universe, but to the internal reality of our ideology opens new avenues to thinking about many of the issues that divide us as a society.

Social constructionism relies on methods of inquiry drawn from symbolic interactionism, symbolic anthropology, ethnomethodology, literary deconstructionism, existentialism, phenomenology, social psychology and other theoretical perspectives that emphasize the role of historical and socio-cultural contingencies in arriving at epistemological assumptions (Tiefer, 1995). In terms of the individual's experience and knowledge of the sexual, social constructionists maintain that our perceptual lenses for seeing the sexual are tinted and framed by a social milieu that is specific to a particular cultural context. "What these disciplines have in common is an emphasis on the person's active role, guided by his or her culture, in structuring the reality that affects his or her own values and behavior" (Tiefer, 1995, p. 18)

Social constructionism emphasizes the cultural origins of the development, substance and meaning of social categories such as masculinity, femininity, heterosexuality, homosexuality, bisexuality, etc. It stresses that sexual meanings and behaviours are learned as culturally normative scripts. "The actual experience of the sexual as well as what is done sexually by individuals is a result of particular learning circumstances of a specific culture" (Gagnon, 1990, p. 4). The record clearly shows that normative patterns of sexual behaviour can change fairly rapidly across both time and place (for a concise review of recent temporal and cross-cultural changes in sexual behaviour see Carballo, Tawil, & Holmes, 1991). Although shifting patterns of sexual behaviour can be multifaceted in origin, these historical and cross-cultural variations in sexual behaviours and beliefs provide credibility to the social constructionist view that sexuality is never free from the guiding hand of ideology.

> When we explore how certain constructs change over time and across cultures, we can start to understand the role of certain groups and organizations in establishing new ideas and expectations. We can begin to ask, "How does the meaning of certain activities change historically?" and "For whose benefit does this operate?" We can examine conflict over language, definitions, policy, and legislation. Whether we are discussing stereotypes about men and women, teenage pregnancy, the emergence of a gay community, or the medical discourse on sexually transmitted diseases, social construction theory acknowledges human agency in sexuality and gender. And it becomes increasingly clear that sexual and gender differences are not simply variations but delineate important dimensions of political activity and conduct. (Irvine, 1990, p. 20)

The role of social forces in shaping our sexual beliefs and behaviours does not, in my view, completely negate the possible contributions of biology in the configuration of human sexuality. It does, however, suggest that the forces of history and culture are omnipresent. For example, it has been proposed that some aspects of human sexual desire, behaviour and even sexual morality are the artifacts of evolutionary processes (Buss, 1994; Symons, 1979; 1980; Wright, 1994). As anthropologist Donald Symons (1980) argues, "Human beings, like all living things, were designed by natural selection. On this there is little scientific question. Natural selection is the only known candidate" (p. 171). Thus, according to Symons and others who argue for a psychobiological explanation of human sexual behaviour, our genetic heritage, moulded by the forces of natural selection, creates psychological predispositions that shape our sexual desires and behaviours. This psychobiological theory of sexuality closely corresponds to the underpinnings of Naturalist sexual ideology and its validity rests on an acceptance of an evolutionary world view and of the power of natural selection to influence our sexuality. It is not my intention here, nor is it necessary, to argue that all aspects of human sexual behaviour are either biologically or socially driven. Rather, I am suggesting that our beliefs, our ideologies related to sexuality, are, to a very great extent, socio-cultural constructions.

In any case, the extent to which this psychobiological perspective corresponds to a hypothetically culture-free human nature is unavoidably muted in its relevance by the mediating powers of the social environment. In the words of Jerome Bruner (1990), "The biological substrate, the so-called universals of human nature, is not a cause of action but, at most, a constraint upon it or a condition for it" (p. 20-21). Most importantly, biology has little or no impact on how we construct and perceive the meaning of sexuality. According to Tiefer (1995), our sexuality is

> a concept with shifting but deeply felt definitions. Conceptualizing sex is a way of corralling and discussing certain human potentials for consciousness, behavior, and expression that are available to be developed by social forces, that is, available to be produced, changed, modified, organized, and defined. Like jell-O, sexuality has no shape without a container, in this case a sociohistorical container of meaning and regulation. (p. 7)

Thus, even our most basic assumptions, as individuals and groups, scientists, theologians, and lay persons, about the nature and purpose of human sexuality can only be confirmed or rejected within the context of a particular version of what must be an admittedly subjective socially constructed reality.

The social constructionist conceptualization of the sexual as being subjectively experienced, through cultural contingencies, extends also to our attempts to discover, through social science inquiry, the nature of human sexuality. As Simon (1989) puts it, "Despite its implicit posture of describing social life from some transcendent elevation, all social science remains inescapably part of the social world it attempts to describe, explain and understand" (p. 32). To the extent that this proposition is accurate, establishing the superiority of one sexual ideology over another with any reasonable degree of certainty becomes highly problematic.

Along with theology, the science of sexology represents our society's most formalized, or official, means of acquiring insights about human sexuality. Sexology, as defined by the American College of Sexology is "the interdisciplinary science of sex including its anatomical, physiological, psychological, medical, sociological, anthropological, historical, legal, religious, literary, and artistic aspects" (Francoeur, Perper, & Scherzer, 1991, p. 588). It is often presumed that science can tell us the unbiased truth about sex. But can sexology maintain a genuine value neutrality?

In our culture, we have often been accustomed to thinking of sharp distinctions between science and philosophy. We commonly think of science as the domain of empirical proof: provider of observable facts. Philosophy, however, is commonly thought of as the domain of belief, perception, reasoned argument, and values. In this view, while a philosophic position may be entirely persuasive, it is, unlike the fact driven scientific stance, a perception or value driven argument. In advancing their theories about the nature of human sexuality, many 20th century sex researchers have striven to portray themselves as investigators employing the methods of empirical science rather than as social philosophers engaging in speculative conjecture.[1] For example, Money (1991) argues that those working in the fields of sexual medicine, therapy, and education are influenced by what he suggests are the conceptually distinct concepts of "sexology" and "sexosophy."

> On the one side of the divide is the sexual researcher; on the other side, the sexual law reformer. To the researcher belongs sexology, the concepts of which derive from the principles of science; to the reformer belongs sexosophy, the concepts of which derive from a philosophy of sexuality. (Money, 1991, p.1)

As Clive Davis (1992) notes, "'sexosophy' seems to smack of bias, of preconceived notions, of values, of subjectivity" (p. 12). And yet, sexosophy seems to continually make its presence felt in the discipline of sexology.

> The positions advocated or opposed by some who call themselves sexologists concerning such controversial issues as sexual addiction, sexually explicit materials, childhood (particularly adult-child) sexual expression, and sexual orientations are by no means objective, supported by empirical evidence; nor are the views of some who advocate particular forms of sexuality education or particular types of sex therapy techniques as *the* right way to do it. These positions and actions are not the result of having reconciled well thought out theoretical perspectives with reliable and valid evidence. These positions are more often based on implicit assumptions and values about the nature of sexuality and what defines good or bad, right or wrong, acceptable or unacceptable sex that have not been validated. (Davis, 1992, p. 13)

Unless these positions are subject to objective validation, Davis' observation suggests that it may be inevitable that sexology and sexosophy must be reconciled as "the two halves of one whole" (Money, cited in Davis, 1992, p. 12).

Any attempt to prove the superiority of a particular sexual ideology must confront the inevitability that our theorizing, whether in terms of scientific or philosophical-religious paradigms, is unavoidably built on the foundation of some basic presuppositions. These presuppositions are, as Reiss (1993) puts it, "the general assumptions we make about how the world operates, including moral assumptions about how it should operate" (p. 4). Drawing from Thomas Kuhn's influential critique of positivistic science in *The Structure of Scientific Revolutions*, Reiss (1993) suggests that what we refer to as "facts" derived from empirical data are themselves dependant in their creation on the paradigmatic presuppositions of the person or group who is making the statement of fact. As a result, these data, and the conclusions drawn from it, "are not a precise representation of the 'true external reality' of the world" (Reiss, 1993, p. 4).

> Kuhn's major point was that to see the world we must make some basic assumptions, what I am calling presuppositions, about how the world operates. We need some presuppositional lenses through which to see the world, or we are blind. We are not born wearing the one correct prescription lens for perceiving reality. Our basic assumptions, or presuppositions, lead us to a theory about how the world operates. What we call empirical data or "facts" are shaped by these prior views of reality. Facts are not just there to be discovered. Rather...we begin to observe a selective set of "facts" only after we start to view the world through the lenses prescribed by our presuppositions. (Reiss, 1993, p. 4)

What becomes immediately apparent here is that ideological and scientific paradigms are fashioned using the same epistemological dynamics. Both require presuppositions that colour the way the world is seen.

In Chapter Two, I suggested that each sexual ideology encompasses particular conceptualizations of the nature of human sexuality, assumptions about sexuality's inherently negative, benign, or positive attributes, and about the function of sexual desire and behaviour which in turn lead to conclusions regarding the naturalness or unnaturalness of specific sexual behaviours. So, for example, within Restrictive sexual ideology sexual pleasure is essentially negative in its character and consequences and the function of sex is reproduction. Behaviours that fall inside this conceptualization are deemed natural and those that fall outside it, such as homosexuality, are condemned as unnatural. In other words, in order to decide if a given sexual behaviour is natural, we must have a standard of nature against which to compare and evaluate the behaviour. But what is nature? We can only discover nature by looking through the lens of our ideological presuppositions about the world.

> What we call natural is, in fact, a confused mixture of biological and religious explanations used to justify our culture's norms. When we label sexual behavior as "natural" or "unnatural" we are actually indicating whether the behavior conforms to our culture's sexual norms. (Strong & Devault, 1994, p. 35)

The use of the terms *nature* or *natural*, however, often functions to mask the subjective, socially constructed basis of what is being said. By employing these terms in our rhetoric "the existence of a material world that lies outside of human intervention is assumed" (Tiefer, 1995, p. 32).

> By emphasizing that something *is in nature*, an author gives whatever is being discussed solidity and validity. That special rhetorical power often seems to call on nature *by contrast with culture*, as if anything human-made can be the result of trickery, but something prior to and outside of human culture can be trusted. The laws of nature, for example, are thought to be above human politics, while the laws of people are polluted with politics. The term confers the authority of something before or underneath culture, something prior to culture. Sexual nature, then, sounds like something solid and valid, not human made. (Tiefer, 1995, pp. 32-33)

Once ideologically bound visions of what is *natural* become embedded within a culture, they take on the appearance of objective truth, a taken-for-granted set of assumptions about the way things really are. The social constructionist analysis of sexuality has helped to bring about an awareness that our perceptions of the nature of sexuality are contained within the confines of ideology. Among the many implications of this new-found awareness is that, evolutionary psychology notwithstanding, many aspects of our sexual nature are culture bound.[2]

> We have recognized that ideology works precisely by making us believe that what is socially created and therefore subjected to change is really natural and therefore inevitable. We no longer believe that of all social phenomena sexuality is the least changeable but, on the contrary, that it is probably the most sensitive to social influence, a conductor of the subtlest changes in social mores and power relations. (Weeks, 1992, p. 393)

In sum, our ideological presuppositions provide the conceptual hook upon which we hang our philosophical beliefs about the nature of the universe and, subsequently, our convictions regarding the naturalness of various sexual behaviours. This, in turn means that, as Habermas (1990) puts it, "an exclusive division of labour between philosophy and science is untenable" (p. 14). Sexosophy and sexology are never completely divisible. Although social scientists conducting research in human sexuality have developed, mainly in the last two decades, sophisticated methods of investigation resulting in increasingly sound theoretical constructs,[3] the emergence of post-positivistic science and postmodern analysis has made rigid truth claims in the social sciences difficult to support (Rosenau, 1992, p. 89).

This scepticism of truth claims helps to explain why the science of sexology, although it may be quite useful in many respects, cannot help us, to any great extent, in resolving ideological disputes about the nature of human sexuality. In the realm of sexuality, ideology and science are never completely separable.

> Consequently, those who attempt to refute, say, the Jehovanist interpretation of sex through "scientific" research will seldom dissuade a single believer, no matter how impeccable their logic or irrefutable their facts. For the world views that underlie sexual interpretations are not held rationally, but rather are the very conditions of rationality. They determine which arguments about a topic seem reasonable and persuasive. Most scientific studies of sex simply do not seem reasonable and persuasive to Jehovanists because they disregard what Jehovanists regard as its most important aspects. Thus Naturalist sexologists "talk past" Jehovanists (and of course Jehovanists do the same to them). (Davis, 1983, p. 230)

The objective validity of our assumptions about the nature of human sexuality must, to some degree, be illusionary and suspect since nothing that we perceive, think, or say can be entirely independent of the social world within which we exist or the ideological space that we occupy. This does not mean that we can never say anything meaningful about sexuality or present compelling, albeit ideologically based, arguments about what is the best approach to sexuality issues. Nor does it mean that the findings of sexologists cannot be helpful in better understanding human sexuality. It does mean that those who claim to know the complete and final truth about such matters, and who claim that others must be made to see this truth, should be viewed with a wary eye.

> Ultimately, there is only one criterion by which beliefs can be judged valid, and that is that they are based on agreement reached by argumentation. This means that *everything* whose validity is at all disputable rests on shaky foundations. It matters little if the ground underfoot shakes a bit less for those who debate problems of physics than for those who debate problems of morals and aesthetics. The difference is a matter of degree only, as the post-empiricist philosophy of science has shown. (Habermas, 1990, p. 14)

If the modern history of sexuality, and the social constructionist tradition in particular, reveals anything that is definitive or indisputable, it is that the foundational ground underneath the discourse on sexuality shakes with the force of an earthquake.

If our ideas about the nature of human sexuality cannot be realistically held up as universalized truths, what about the ethics that various ideologies propose to guide sexual behaviour? Are we able to make axiomatic claims about the relative merits of ideological conceptualizations of right and wrong sexual behaviour? As we begin to lay the foundations for social policy around sexuality related issues, including a philosophy to guide sexuality education in the schools, this question becomes of fundamental importance.

Within the realm of Restrictive and Permissive sexual ideologies, their respective claims about the nature of sexuality and the ethics that ought to govern sexual behaviour are one and the same theory extended in different directions. If sex is, from the Restrictive perspective, essentially negative in nature, it follows that the moral rules that govern it should direct sexual behaviour in the direction of its narrow range of socially desirable outcomes: procreation and/or intimacy in "mature," monogamous relationships. If sex is, from the Permissive perspective, either benign or positive in nature, it follows that the moral rules that govern it should allow for a wide range of contexts in which sexual acts are morally acceptable.

This is not to suggest that universal moral principles of human conduct cannot be identified or justified, but rather that since the sexual ethics proposed by Restrictive and Permissive sexual ideology derive part of their justification from socially constructed notions about the nature of human sexuality that constitute truth only for those who share that ideological world view, neither moral paradigm has universal applicability. For those who do not inhabit the ideological space of a particular sexual ideology, reconciling that ideology's concept of sexual morality as representative of objective morality is a non-starter. It is akin to being asked to see an apple as an orange. As Fromer (1983) puts it "To be universalizable, a moral theory must be sufficiently concrete to be understood by a vast majority of rational people" (pp. 2-3). In regards to the specific criteria used to judge the morality of particular sexual acts, the adherents of opposing sexual ideologies do not share a concrete common ground. This is why those with a Restrictive sexual ideology cannot accept the epistemological foundations of person-centred sexual ethics and why those with a Permissive sexual ideology cannot endorse the logic of an act-centred sexual ethics.

As I discussed in Chapters One and Two, particularly in relation to the development of Restrictive sexual ideology, many of our prevailing beliefs about sexuality are religious in origin. Therefore, we need to consider, at least briefly, the ideological claims about sexual morality that are rooted in theological interpretations of sexuality. Although religious traditions consist of both concrete socio-cultural and abstract spiritual elements (Progoff, 1963), when regarded as systems of spiritual belief, the claim on behalf of a particular religious tradition for the universal application of that tradition's sexual ethics is subject to the same problems faced by secular moral truth claims.

It perhaps goes without saying that, at their very essence, religious beliefs are a matter of faith rather than of concrete observations about the material world. Faith "is based on the religious experience of people as they individually relate to the transcendent" (Johnstone, 1975, p. 14). And subsequently, the individual's relationship with the transcendent involves an element of the "supernatural, a power or being not subject to the laws of the observable universe" (Johnstone, 1975, pp. 16-17). In the moral domain, ethics based on religious faith require "human beings to make some response to God....A theistic orientation must relate to moral ideas or there would be no point to theologic theories of morality" (Fromer, 1983, p. 31).

> A logical relation implies that a practice derives from a belief and that a particular belief implies a practice. A psychologic relation denotes that a theistic orientation motivates obligations or duties, that is, reasons for developing one's character in certain ways or for doing certain actions arise from a theistic orientation. An epistomologic relation implies that one *can* know that a theistic orientation contrib-

utes to morality. This relation holds that certain truths are known *only* through a theistic orientation. The ontologic relation holds that the existence of moral obligation is vitally connected with the existence and activity of God. If everything in existence depends on the existence of God, then morality also depends on the existence of God. (Fromer, 1983, p. 32)

In this sense, the epistemological foundation upon which spiritual beliefs are grounded represents the foundation for moral truth only in so far as one accepts, on the basis of faith (i.e., knowing God), that which cannot be comprehended in a concrete, directly observable context. Put another way, the world view and essence of religious beliefs, including moral truths, are given form and transmitted to us through symbolization. That is, "religions exist in symbolic forms" (Spinks, 1963, p. 68).

Although some of the adherents of the various religious faiths believe that their particular religious text (i.e., The Bible, The Koran, The Torah) must be interpreted literally as sacred infallible truth, this claim is itself dependent on a faith, a particular set of strongly held spiritual beliefs that is infallible only to those that share the ideological reality of the religion in question. To see The Bible, for example, as a source of unimpeachable moral rules for sexual conduct makes sense only to those who have faith in the sacred authority of The Bible.

In sum, there are multiple, and widely divergent, avenues to discovering the truth about sexuality. When the theologian interprets scripture and the sexologist interprets empirical research data, they are each revealing a truth which will make sense to those individuals and groups within society that share the ideological perspective of the theologian or the sexologist. With respect to sexual morality, no philosopher is likely to convince all, or even a stable majority, of us that a particular moral theory of sexual conduct is objectively correct. Without being flippant about the issue, to use the words of Fromer (1983)

It is obvious to any aware reader that no ethicist or moral philosopher from Socrates to the present has presented conclusive proof, to the satisfaction of all thinkers, that one moral theory is superior to all others. (p. 13)

Whether or not the truth about sexuality, in an objective sense, is ultimately identifiable is somewhat of a moot point. For the true believers in various sexual ideologies, the truth about sex is already self-evident. But this brand of truth is located in the subjective paradigms of ideological belief systems which are themselves subject to enormous variation. Thus, we need to understand individual and group beliefs about the sexual within the context of their culturally situated sexual ideology that serves as the foundation for arriving at a socially constructed truth in sexual matters. This does not imply

> an abandonment of all we have learned about the constancies and varieties of the biological substratum, but it does require the effort of going beyond that and examining that which can only be understood in terms of individuals situated in specific points of social space and specific points in time; individuals with and within history. (Simon, 1989, p. 23)

Implications for Contemporary Sexuality Education

The social constructionist analysis of sexuality has, in the words of Naus and Theis (1991),

> far-reaching consequences for sex education and sex therapy. Most importantly, it raises questions about the objectives or desired outcomes of these practices, and about the manner in which these objectives are decided upon. The objectives are usually derived from explicit or implicit concepts of what sexuality really is, and the development of these concepts, as well as the derivation of objectives from them, are typically done by experts, that is, by individuals who claim scientific or professional expertise about sexuality. (p. 20)

Among other things, Naus and Theis (1991) argue that the social constructionist analysis of sexuality strongly suggests that the objectives for sexuality education "reflect the diversity of constructed sexuality and emphasize that people need the freedom to make their own sexual choices" (p. 20).

How well do the three currently predominant variations of sexuality education in the schools, described in Chapter Three, meet the standard set by Naus and Theis? In other words, do sexuality education programs that are reflective of Restrictive or Permissive sexual ideology or the barebones approach adequately address the diversity of constructed sexuality and provide students with the freedom to make choices congruent with their own ideological perspectives?

In the case of sexuality education that is largely informed by either Restrictive or Permissive sexual ideology, the answer is clear. As we have seen, these types of sexuality education are exclusively partial in their approach to sexual morality, precluding an even or balanced presentation of divergent ideological perspectives toward sexuality. Thus, it is extremely unlikely that such programs can realistically reflect the existing diversity of constructed sexuality within Western society because they tend to address sexuality issues from a particular ideological perspective without a complimentary consideration of alternative perspectives. Further, without such a complimentary consideration of alternative perspectives, it is also highly unlikely that such programs are conducive to students making their own choices. Within the intellectual climate of the classroom, choices that are congruent with the preferred sexual ideology are inevitably encouraged at least implicitly if not explicitly.

The bare-bones approach to sexuality education also fails to meet the standards set out by Naus and Theis. It is difficult to see how sexuality education can adequately reflect the diversity of constructed sexuality in our society if educational programs are designed to avoid the often divisive issues that are the product of ideological diversity. Bare-bones sexuality education, with its exclusively neutral tendency, is unlikely to stimulate students' capacity to think critically about important social issues related to sexuality. To deliberately circumvent the opportunity for students to address such issues is questionable by all but the most totalitarian of standards. The problematic nature of a position of exclusive neutrality is summed up by Kelly (1986) when he writes that schools,

> particularly those publically financed and state supported in a democracy, have a moral responsibility to develop in their charges the understandings, competencies and commitments to be effective citizens. Among other attributes, these broad goals include the ability to make informed judgements in a reasoned, if passionate manner. In order to achieve these democratic goals, teachers need to include rather than exclude public controversy. (p. 114)

In addition, as we saw in Chapter One, it is now widely recognized by a large majority of people that sexuality education in the schools serves a useful purpose. The importance of sexuality education is most often associated with the desire to help teenagers avoid unintended pregnancy and sexually transmitted diseases including HIV/AIDS. There is considerable evidence to suggest that bare-bones sexuality education is of little value in this respect. Evaluations of the behavioural effects of sexuality education programs implemented during the 1970s and 1980s show that these programs, more often than not, did nothing to help teenagers protect their sexual health (e.g., Kirby, 1984; Stout & Rivera, 1989). The primary reason for this, according to many researchers, is that these programs excluded the necessary information and skills for adolescents to either abstain from intercourse or practise safer sex (see Brown & Eisenberg, 1995, pp. 131-135; Kirby et al, 1994). Brown and Eisenberg (1995) conclude from their review of studies on the content of school-based sexuality education that programs are characterized by "a lack of prevention information" (p. 133). As Brown and Eisenberg (1995) state,

> While it is true that many states require schools to provide sexuality education and HIV/AIDS education to students at different grade levels, it is also the case that in many states, the content of those educational programs is limited by statute or by state policy or both (The Alan Guttmacher Institute, 1989). The precise nature of these restrictions can serve to limit the effectiveness of the educational programs by, for example, prohibiting explicit discussion of topics directly related to pregnancy prevention, such as contraception. (p. 132)

As Nicolas Freudenberg (1989) aptly puts it in discussing the social and political obstacles to effective HIV/AIDS prevention education, "The danger of education that offends no one is that it may fail in its effort to communicate anything at all to those most in need of the information and resources at the time" (p. 3). In sum, the bare-bones approach to sexuality education is unacceptable from a health perspective because in seeking to avoid controversy it is bound to omit the information and skills necessary for students to protect their sexual health.

Aside from issues related specifically to physical health, sexuality, as we have seen is deeply imbued with personal and social significance. Few would disagree with the view that our psychological well-being is inherently interconnected with our sexuality. In other words, successfully meeting the developmental challenges that sexuality presents us with throughout our lifetimes is an important factor in determining our overall health and well-being. We can likely agree that education might help us to meet this challenge by, at the very least, providing a solid knowledge base upon which to gain a basic understanding of sexuality. This being the case, a bare-bones approach to sexuality education is likely to be of little value in this respect.

While the bare-bones approach to sexuality education offers the highly desired avoidance of public controversy, it is clearly a deficient solution to the ideological struggle over the form and content of sexuality education in the schools. In order to arrive at a just and workable solution to this dilemma we must deepen our understanding of the nature of sexual ideology and its place in a democratic society.

Conclusion

If the solution to the dilemma of conflicting sexual ideologies cannot be found through an epistemological consensus on what constitutes an objectively superior sexual morality, we then have no alternative but to turn to a pragmatic or political solution to the conflict of sexual ideologies. This, however, does not imply that sexuality must become a moral-free zone. Rather it suggests that the moral dimension of the solution rests at a higher political level than at the level of specific disagreements around ideologically laden issues of sexuality. In other words, the problem of conflicting sexual ideologies is a type of problem that is specific to democratic societies where a multiplicity of ideologies are permitted to exist. In this sense, in a democratic society our moral imperative is not to establish which ideology is correct, but rather "moral thinking is essentially thinking about the fundamental values by which we profess to live" (Duncan, 1979, p. 7). As I shall propose in the next chapter, these higher order fundamental values of democracy provide a means of mediating between sexual ideologies in a way that preserves their integrity while at the same time allowing, as is consistent with a democratic society, a pluralism of ideologies to coexist. Subsequently, a democratic philosophy of education can be explored as a means of mediating ideological conflict around sexuality education.

Notes

1.   For historical accounts of the methodologies of modern sexology see Bullough, 1994; Irvine, 1990; Robinson, 1977.

2.   This point should not be taken to mean that the Restrictive ideological belief in a fixed view of human nature is any less correct than the Permissive ideological belief in an evolving view of human nature. Rather, it suggests that all beliefs in particular visions of human nature are to some extent culture bound. As Weeks (1995) notes, "Social constructionism has no political belonging. It does not carry with it any obvious programme. On

the contrary, it can be, and has been, used recently as much by sexual conservatives as by sexual progressives" (p. 8).

Restrictive ideological approaches to homosexuality offer a clear example of the social constructionist bent of some Restrictive ideological thinking. For example, Jehovanist ideologues do not deny that homosexual desire exists or that culture has shaped and, much to their consternation, legitimized homosexual identities. Indeed, their approach is profoundly constructionist in that they believe that if moral and legal prohibitions against homosexuality are applied rigorously and consistently enough, the practice of homosexual behaviour will be greatly diminished if not eliminated. The fact that many Restrictive ideologues argue for a sexual morality based on the presumably objective standards of God's commandments does not logically prevent them from invoking a social constructionist analysis of sexuality. They acknowledge the social and historical relativity of human affairs but see it as opening up the possibilities for humanity to drift away from God's will. The solution for the Restrictive ideologue is to aggressively pursue social norms that bring us as close as possible to the infallible objective moral standards of the supernatural.

3.   For a review of contemporary sexological theory see Geer and O'Donohue, 1987.

CHAPTER FIVE

Sexuality, Moral Pluralism, and the Concept of Liberal Democracy

▬ ·· ▬ ·· ▬ ▬ ·· ▬ ·· ▬ ▬ ·· ▬ ·· ▬ ▬ ·· ▬ ·· ▬ ·· ▬ ··

> The contemporary sexual world appears as irrevocably pluralistic, divided into a host of sovereign units, and a multiplicity of sites of authority, none of which claim a firm foundation. There is no longer a hegemonic master discourse telling how we should behave, and those clamant moralities which attempt to fill the vacuum may have their listeners, but cannot affirm an ultimate legitimacy.
>
> (Weeks, 1995)

> One sign of a healthy Western civilization is that within a relatively integrated moral outlook—for example, agreement on democratic principles—a myriad of ideas and methods are brought face to face. Through civilized conflict the society's assumed moral correctness is constantly tested. This tension—emotional, intellectual, moral—is what advances the society.
>
> (Saul, 1993)

Introduction

The social and political dilemmas facing us in Western democracies are many and perplexing. As contrasted with totalitarian societies, moral issues and social policy are the subject of never ending debate in the Western democracies. It is the clash of freely articulated ideas and perspectives in reasoned debate that provides the framework for the making of presumably enlightened social policy. The deliberative process is the heart, for example, of the parliamentary system. With respect to the individual, democracy endows us with the right to moral autonomy but this autonomy is genuine only when we are free to digest diverse or opposing perspectives in reaching our own point of view. Providing this opportunity to deliberate between competing points of view pervades a democratic way of life. Perpetually accommodating and deliberating between conflicting points of view is the happy fate of living in a society characterized by liberty, moral pluralism and, presumably, equal respect for the rights of all persons. However, confronted by strongly held but unprovable social-political "truths" and opposing wills, we are left only with our most fundamental, and hopefully shared, values and principles as a means of resolving our differences.

Contemporary Western societies are constitutionally conceived as liberal democracies. However, as Giroux and Maclaren (1992) point out "Consistently, the notion of democracy is invoked as an inviolable principle but rarely defined as a social or cultural practice" (p. xi). If we begin to think of the constitutive elements of democracy as a social or cultural practice we begin, I believe, with the idea of freedom of belief. Accorded with freedom of belief, each of us is provided at least with the possibility of autonomously choosing our own conception of the good life. The first two "fundamental freedoms" accorded to all citizens of Canada in the *Canadian Charter of Rights and Freedoms* are " (a) freedom of conscience and religion; (b) freedom of thought, belief, opinion and expression" (*Canadian Charter of Rights and Freedoms*, Appendix B in Gosh & Ray, 1987, p. 281). The constitutions of other Western liberal democracies, particularly the United States, place freedom of conscience, religion, and belief at the core of the commonly shared national ethos.

Freedom of belief is held not only to protect the individual's right to autonomously choose a conception of the good life, but also to foster the development of intellect and wisdom that advances and perpetuates a democratic culture. As John Dewey observes about democracy in the United States,

> the basic freedom of action and experience is necessary to produce freedom of intelligence. The modes of freedom guaranteed in the Bill of Rights are all of this nature: Freedom of belief and conscience, of expression of opinion, of assembly for discussion and conference, of the press as an organ of communication. They are guaranteed because without them individuals are not free to develop and society is deprived of what they might contribute. (Dewey cited in Mosher, Kenny, and Garrod, 1994, p. 35)

An exclusive focus on the freedom of conscience, religion, and belief is, of course, too simplistic a summation to characterize realistically the intricacies of a liberal democratic society, but I do believe it captures its most essential element, particularly when liberal democracy is contrasted to totalitarianism. Although democracy is a wide ranging and complex concept, I am focussing here on those elements of it related specifically to the freedom of belief, conscience, and the freedom to form beliefs through the process of unencumbered critical deliberation. I take it as a basic, and hopefully realistic, assumption that those who consent to citizenship in a democratic state endorse these freedoms as indispensable to a just society. In articulating a philosophy of sexuality education based on democratic principles, I will emphasize the principle of freedom of belief because I believe that this principle is at the very foundation of a democratic society and that the opportunity to deliberate between divergent points of view is *the* central constitutive element of a democratic education.

The most obvious and complicating factor related to the basic freedoms of liberal democracy is that these freedoms can often collide, resulting in a situation where one person's or group's freedom places a significant burden on another person's or group's freedom. As a result, the basic freedoms inherent in liberal democracy are not absolute. They are limited by the obligation to respect the equal right of others to these same freedoms. Such obligations are, for example, expressed through democratic precepts such as the principle of nondiscrimination. The struggle to effectively balance the right to freedom of belief with the equally important right to live a life free of discrimination is at the centre of democratic discourse. This delicate balancing of fundamental but often conflicting rights must, as much as possible, be unambiguously understood and practised with great care if genuine democracy is to prevail. From the onset, then, we must make clear that the right to hold a given moral belief does not translate into a complementary right to try to impose that belief on others or on society at large. The failure to make this distinction adequately, frequently rears its ugly head in the Western cultural discourse on sexuality. For example, an individual does, within a democracy, have the right to disapprove morally of homosexual behaviour. The right to hold such a belief cannot, however, serve to justify a belief in the legitamcy of attempting to curtail the rights of homosexuals. Within a democracy, the former does not logically extend to the latter. In Western culture these two beliefs have often been conflated and the result has been rampant discrimination.

Thus, among the central tasks of the public institutions of liberal democracies is to balance conflicting freedoms in a fair and equitable fashion. In essence, this comes down to the delicate exercise of accommodating different and often opposing claims, points of view, and values. As Moon (1993) suggests, "The commitment to accommodating difference is at the heart of political liberalism" (p. 191). As I shall suggest, acknowledgement of the basic democratic task of accommodating difference has profound implications for sexuality education in particular and social policy related to sexuality in general. It is necessary first, however, to place the dilemma of Western society's plurality of sexual ideologies in the context of a democratic framework for accommodating moral differences. I do acknowledge that the meaning of democracy is, as it should be, up for debate and that it is the subject of varying interpretations. In this chapter, I will therefore outline what I strongly believe to be the essential unifying principles of liberal democracy. These principles are those basic values and conventions that are presumably shared by all people who willingly consent to live by the rules of a democratic regime. In order to accomplish this task I will rely almost entirely on philosopher John Rawls' (1993) *Political Liberalism* which I believe reasonably articulates the essential elements of liberal democracy.

The argument that the elemental features of a democratic society can be deduced from the theory of political liberalism will be contested by some. A conservative conception of democracy will draw much more heavily on the need to preserve the established social traditions which have allowed democracies to flourish in the first place. While generally not hostile to the concept of individual liberty, particularly in economic matters, conservatives argue for the need to balance individual liberties with a much stronger emphasis than most liberals would like on preserving established practices that have played a role in defining and ordering society. From this conservative point of view, disturbing the norms of traditional morality is inherently destructive. The moral traditions of Western culture bind together and maintain our society.

I do not want to dismiss the conservative notion that the character of democratic culture is, at least in part, built and maintained on the preservation of certain political, economic, and social traditions. However, I do want to argue quite strongly that there are fundamental and inescapable problems associated with an argument that the importance of preserving the established practices of Western culture can logically be extended to justify enforcing some of our most highly contested moral and political traditions related to sexuality. The preservation of tradition cannot, in a democratic society, come at the expense of our most fundamental rights and freedoms. By its very nature, a truly democratic society is not intransigently resistant to even fundamental modifications to some of its established social, legal, and political practices. The abolition of slavery and the advent of universal suffrage are prime examples of how such modifications enhance, not detract from, the democratic character of society.

Closely aligned with the conservative conception of democracy is the communitarian view that the values and traditions of a particular community can rightly be promoted in contrast to the values or social traditions of the larger society. Community leaders who explicitly state and promote the values and traditions that are held to define the community are not necessarily at odds with the larger liberal state. However, in a liberal democracy there are limits to the degree to which values of a particular community can be promoted. Where communitarianism silences or excludes the expression of other or even clearly dissenting views, the principles of liberal democracy have been violated. This is a particularly salient issue with respect to sexuality and sexuality education. As Middleman (1996) points out, an extreme form of communitarianism can negatively impact on the right to knowledge about sexuality and of freedom of belief.

> Each community defines its own rules regarding sex, sexuality, what can be taught in schools, and what restrictions on information can exist. It is in the communitarian society that the community may decide the rules of the society, regardless of individual rights. Thus, if a religious community, for example, would like to prevent sexuality education in the schools, that is the prerogative of the community. (p. 306)

This communitarian perspective has been used as a justification to impose sexual ideology in the schools. In terms of individual rights, this application of communitarian values is clearly at odds with the basic tenets of a liberal democracy. As Middleman (1996) notes, we live in a society that is at its most fundamental level liberal, not communitarian. Western constitutions do not contain provisions allowing communities to over-ride basic individual rights.

A unified truth about sexuality eludes us and because we live in a highly heterogeneous society, from a sociological perspective, we will likely live in a society with multiple versions of sexual truth for the foreseeable future.

> In complex societies such cultural scenarios for sexuality are not monolithic or hegemonic, even within institutions. Instead there is a

> constant struggle between groups and individuals to foster their own
> scenarios. Some are more powerful than others, but no individual or
> group or institution is in entire control of the sexual scenarios for most
> Western societies. (Gagnon, 1990, p. 9)

As a result there is "an emergent consensus about the absence of consensus.
And perhaps, not so much an absence of consensus but a sense of being
forced to an unexpected and often discomforting pluralism" (Simon, 1989,
pp. 18-19). Given the existence of a pluralism of sexual ideologies and their
corresponding moral truths, the identification of, and consensus for, a
normative sexual ethics—moral principles related to sexuality that all
people can and ought to be guided by—is unlikely to be within our grasp.

In the case of sexuality, a simple reliance on tradition to guide us is
unworkable since the all-encompassing hegemonic position of Restrictive
sexual ideology is irretrievably in the past. This tradition is ever increasingly
contested by so many and it is neither applicable nor valid for large segments
of Western society. With respect to moral pluralism, analogies can be drawn
between sexuality and the democratic freedoms of religion and expression.
They are all crucial to an individual's self-determination and self-definition,
fundamental pathways to the good life in any conception of democracy.
Karen Struening (1995) suggests that

> We value and protect the freedoms of religion and expression, in part,
> because we believe that wrestling with and coming to our own religious
> and moral judgements is an essential component of self-determination
> and self-definition. The freedoms of sexual choice and intimate asso-
> ciation play an analogous role in the individual's life....The regulation
> and repression of noncoercive and consensual sexual practices be-
> tween adults is a direct assault on moral pluralism. It is as serious an
> abridgement of personal liberty as efforts to curtail the freedoms of
> religion and expression. (pp. 508-509)

In the absence of a master ideology stipulating the sexually good life,
imposing the traditions of the past on those who find them disagreeable or
dysfunctional is to interfere, in a very fundamental way, with the most basic
of democratic rights.

Because human beings are social animals who do not live in isolation
from each other but must live together in a multiplicity of social relationships, we cannot leave the issue of opposing sexual ideologies at the point
of a simple "agree to disagree" relativism. Issues such as the form and

content of the sexuality education of youth are not resolved by an uncomplicated acknowledgement that we, as a society, cannot realistically hope
to come to an agreement on which sexual ideology should inform educational programs in the public schools. Such an acknowledgement is a
necessary step on our way to identifying an adequate philosophy of sexuality
education, but it is by itself insufficient. We must go beyond this to explore
how, in a society characterized by a diversity of sexual ideologies, sexuality
education in the schools can, in a reasonable, fair, and constructive manner,
contribute to the socialization of youth so that it reflects the interests and
needs of the individual and his/her peer group, family, community, religious-
ethnocultural tradition, and society as a whole. All of these groups have
something at stake when the form and content of sexuality education in the
schools is established. In order to proceed with this line of inquiry we need
to step back, at least for a while, from addressing specific issues of disagreement (i.e., the morality of teenage sex, homosexuality, etc.) and examine
the larger issue of how our society can accommodate a pluralism of often
conflicting sexual ideologies. We need to grasp the opportunity, as Weeks
(1992) suggests,

> to reinvent or rediscover values that help us to live with what seems
> to me the only irreducible truth of the contemporary world: the fact
> of human and social diversity, including sexual diversity. This is the
> real challenge of living with uncertainty. (p. 393)

As Rawls (1993) puts it, "This is a problem of political justice, not a problem
about the highest good" (p. xxv).

Political Liberalism

In *Political Liberalism*, Rawls (1993) explores how, in a democratic
society, the concept of political liberalism can provide an overarching
political framework that is consistent with the ideals or "very great values"
of democracy. When we, as ideologues of all reasonable stripes, are willing
to commit to this overarching framework, we reach, according to Rawls, an
"overlapping consensus" which serves to allow people with different and
opposing beliefs to live together in a free and democratic society and yet
maintain the integrity of our respective beliefs.

In *Political Liberalism*, Rawls (1993) uses the term *comprehensive doctrines*
to demarcate different and opposing belief systems. Comprehensive doc-

trines are roughly analogous to ideologies, in that comprehensive doctrines entail

> conceptions of what is of value in human life, and ideals of personal
> character, as well as ideals of friendship and of familial and associa-
> tional relationships, and much else that is to inform our conduct, and
> in the limit to our life as a whole. A conception is fully comprehensive
> if it covers all recognized values and virtues within one rather precisely
> articulated system; whereas a conception is only partially comprehen-
> sive when it comprises a number of, but by no means all, nonpolitical
> values and virtues and is rather loosely articulated. (Rawls, 1993, p.
> 13)

Within this schema, sexual ideologies tend to constitute a component of a comprehensive doctrine. That is, as we have seen, beliefs about sexuality, including the moral domain, are often part of a wider ideological view of the world. Nonetheless, the central problem facing a democratic society, where social and political life is based on the principles of justice (i.e., liberty, fairness, equality), freedom of belief and the liberty to follow a conception of the good life consistent with those beliefs so long as they do not abrogate these principles, is the same whether we are considering comprehensive doctrines in general or sexual ideologies in particular. Rawls (1993) states the problem and indicates the basic approach to it taken by political liberalism.

> A modern democratic society is characterized not simply by a pluralism
> of comprehensive religious, philosophical, and moral doctrines but by
> a pluralism of incompatible yet reasonable comprehensive doctrines.
> No one of these doctrines is affirmed by citizens generally. Nor should
> one expect in the foreseeable future one of them, or some other
> reasonable doctrine, will ever be affirmed by all, or nearly all, citizens.
> Political liberalism assumes that, for political purposes, a plurality of
> reasonable yet incompatible comprehensive doctrines is the normal
> result of the exercise of human reason within a framework of free
> institutions of a constitutional democratic regime. Political liberalism
> also supposes that a reasonable comprehensive doctrine does not reject
> the essentials of a democratic regime. (Rawls, 1993, p. xvi)

A doctrine is considered reasonable, according to this view, because it acknowledges the right of all persons, no matter what their ideology, to enjoy the rights and freedoms of a democratic society including the freedom of belief. So, for example, the attempt by the adherents of a particular sexual ideology to force their beliefs on others or society as a whole is in conflict with the essentials of a democratic regime. A political conception of justice supports democratic living in that it affirms and mediates between opposing philosophical beliefs.

Briefly, the political conception of justice is defined by its three characteristic features, each of which contributes to a basic conception of justice as fairness. The first feature is the political nature of this conception of justice. That is, it applies to "the 'basic structure' of society, which for our present purposes I take to be a modern constitutional democracy" (Rawls, 1993, p. 11).

> The initial focus, then, of a political conception of justice is the framework of basic institutions and the principles, standards, and precepts that apply to it, as well as how those norms are to be expressed in the character and attitudes of the members of society who realize its ideals. (Ibid., pp. 11-12)

The second feature of a political conception of justice is that it is "presented as a freestanding view" (Ibid., p. 12). That is, the political conception of justice is derived from the shared fundamental values upon which democracy is based. It is not derived from a particular comprehensive doctrine, or in this case, sexual ideology. In this sense, a political conception of justice is conceived of as apart from, although hopefully not in conflict with, a particular ideology.

The third feature of a political conception of justice is that it is expressed in terms of the fundamental social ideals implicit in the public culture of a democratic society.

> comprehensive doctrines of all kinds—religious, philosophical, and moral—belong to what we may call the "background culture" of civil society. This is the culture of the social, not of the political....In a democratic society there is a tradition of democratic thought, the content of which is at least familiar and intelligible to the educated common sense of citizens generally. Society's main institutions, and their accepted forms of interpretation, are seen as a fund of implicitly shared ideas and principles. (Ibid., p. 14)

It is on the basis of this political conception of justice, and our affirmation of it, that the overlapping consensus of political liberalism is achieved.

> Such a consensus consists of all the reasonable opposing religious, philosophical, and moral doctrines likely to persist over generations

and to gain a sizable body of adherents in a more or less just constitutional regime, a regime in which the criterion of justice is that political
conception itself. (Ibid., p. 15)

Are the Restrictive and Permissive sexual ideologies amenable to an
overlapping consensus based on a political conception of justice? The
answer can be affirmative to the extent that

> citizens themselves, within the exercise of their liberty of thought and
> conscience, and looking to their comprehensive doctrines, view the
> political conception as derived from, or congruent with, or at least not
> in conflict with, their other values. (Rawls, 1993, p. 11)

Each ideology must respect the core values of democracy. It must not
call for the coercive imposition of a particular vision of sexuality.[1] In other
words, the proponents of a particular sexual ideology, regardless of whether
it is Restrictive or Permissive, violate the spirit of democracy when they
successfully implement public school-based sexuality education programs
embodying only that ideology. The same principle holds true for other
public institutions such as the legislative and legal systems which must
constantly grapple with sexuality issues. It must, however, be continually
re-emphasized that the overlapping consensus of a liberal democracy does
not preclude the adherents of particular sexual ideologies from presenting
their case to society or engaging in dialogue intended to win new adherents,
provided, of course, that the dialogue between sexual ideologies is fair and
equal.

In *Political Liberalism*, Rawls (1993) presents a detailed account of the
structure and content of the overlapping consensus that allows deeply
opposed belief systems to, more or less, peacefully coexist within the political
structures of a democratic regime. I will focus, here, on those components
of Rawls' framework that are immediately relevant to the issue of conflicting
sexual ideologies and how those components may provide an initial justification for looking towards a democratic philosophy of education as a means
of identifying an overlapping consensus on the sexuality education of youth
in the schools.

In regards to the question of which sexual ideology is superior, the issue
over which most of the ideological battles over sexuality have been fought,
Rawls' conception of political liberalism suggests, as one of its fundamental
principles, that the attempt to verify, once and for all, the claims of particular

ideologies as they pertain to such things as ideals of personal character and the values that guide these ideals, misses the point and purpose of democracy. We saw that the social constructionist perspective on sexuality shows that the truth of sex is available only through ideological lenses and I have suggested that this presents not just an epistemological problem but a political problem as well, leading us to the dilemma of how to shape the form and content of sexuality education. The view of political liberalism, in regard to such questions, is compatible with my analysis of sexual belief systems in that it suggests that a democratic society, with multiple ideologies, is unlikely to arrive at an agreed upon irrefutable "objective" truth in moral matters. In any case, it is not appropriate within a liberal democracy to impose even an objective truth or, as is more likely the case, a particular version of the truth. Political liberalism does not deny ideologies their versions of the truth as being valid within their ideological world views. But neither does it see any of them as the uniform foundation of a democratic society. Political liberalism sees only the basic principles of the commonly agreed to overlapping consensus as democratic society's foundation.

> Political liberalism does not attack or criticize any reasonable view. As a part of this, it does not criticize, much less reject, any particular theory of the truth of moral judgements. In this regard, it simply supposes that judgements of such truth are made from the point of view of some comprehensive moral doctrine....Which moral judgements are true, all things considered is not a matter for political liberalism, as it approaches all questions from within its own limited point of view. (Rawls, 1993, pp. xix-xx)

Following this line of reasoning, there is justification for the assertion that since, as we have seen from the social constructionist analysis, any search for the "truth" about sexuality is unavoidably linked to ideology, in a democratic society social policy, including sexuality education policies, ought to be made from a point of view consistent with the overlapping consensus of political liberalism. In other words, when faced with radically opposing points of view on issues such as sexuality, we must turn to those few commonly held principles that bind us together as a society.

To the ideologues of sex, the affirmation of a pluralism of sexual ideologies has not been an appealing idea. The growth or persistence of one ideology is often seen as intolerable to the other. When examined in the light of a basic democratic ethos, this tendency on the part of those who adhere to a given sexual ideology to seek or favour the obliteration of other ideologies that they do not like partially reveals the destructive, and ultimately undemocratic, nature of the contemporary sexuality debates. Within a liberal democracy, ideological pluralism is actively affirmed, or at the very least tolerated, but certainly not rejected by those who consent to democratic citizenship and who support democratic public institutions.

> This pluralism is not seen as disaster but rather as the natural outcome of the activities of human reason under enduring free institutions. To see reasonable pluralism as a disaster is to see the exercise of reason under the conditions of freedom itself as a disaster. Indeed, the success of liberal constitutionalism came as a discovery of a new social possibility: the possibility of a reasonably harmonious and stable pluralist society. (Ibid., pp. xxiv-xxv)

It might be objected that the exercise of reason under the conditions of freedom is fundamentally in conflict with Restrictive sexual ideology which is seen as relying more on faith and obedience to moral absolutes than it does on an individual's free exercise of reasoned deliberation. However, with respect to sexual ideologies, as I have conceptualized them, the demand for the exercise of reason under the conditions of freedom refers only to individuals being given the opportunity to exercise their reason in the process of developing their ideological perspective. This demand does not, however, set the ground rules for ethical decision making from within the world view of the critically appropriated sexual ideology.

The way in which a society based on liberal democratic principles properly addresses the issue of the relation between the demand for the exercise of reason under the conditions of freedom and its implications for the way each ideology deals with sexual morality can be clarified by making a distinction between what may be called *lower order* and *higher order* ethical issues. Lower order issues relate to the substance of particular questions of sexual morality. How do I, as an individual, know if a particular sexual behaviour is right or wrong? As has been shown, this type of question is inevitably answered through the lens of sexual ideology. Our individual and communal socialization, including our education, provides each of us with an ideological framework that enables us to conceptually organize and answer this type of question. Lower order issues, then, relate to specific questions of sexual morality and the sexual ethics we employ to answer them. They fall within the realm of comprehensive doctrines. That is, lower order issues relate to the specifics of how particular sexual ideologies answer moral questions. Political liberalism has little or no interest in how each sexual ideology answers these questions. For example, political liberalism is not concerned with the question of whether premarital sex is always immoral or not. That is a question for which each sexual ideology has an answer.

Higher order issues are categorically distinct from lower order issues. Higher order issues relate to how the public institutions of the liberal democratic state fairly accommodate a diversity of sexual ideologies, each with its own set of lower order perspectives, in a manner that is consistent with the overlapping consensus. In other words, higher order issues relate to the limited regulative function of political liberalism. Higher order issues are concerned only with creating and maintaining a political and social environment that affords us the freedom to deliberate between divergent ideological perspectives. To use party politics as an analogy, political liberalism is not interested in dictating a political party's policy platform. This is a lower order issue. Rather, political liberalism is interested only in preserving the right of individuals to exercise their reason under the conditions of freedom to deliberate between different party platforms in making the choice of which party to vote for. This is a higher order issue. With respect to sexual ideology, political liberalism is interested in higher order, but not lower order, issues. To return to the example of premarital sex, it is a higher order issue only insofar as people are permitted the freedom to deliberate between different points of view in drawing their own conclusions about whether or not premarital sex is immoral.

The overlapping consensus of political liberalism implies something quite different than does the incorporation of liberal ethics by Permissive sexual ideology. The adoption of the ethics of the secular liberal tradition by Permissive sexual ideology constitutes an element of the broader ideology. Where this ideology, including its specific guidelines for the moral evaluation of sexual behaviour, is imposed on citizens it constitutes an unreasonable doctrine. Political liberalism makes no judgements about the morality of specific forms of sexual belief and behaviour except to say that within a democratic society, individuals and groups must respect the rights and freedoms of those who take a different position. Political liberalism does not endorse Permissive sexual ideology any more than it endorses Restrictive sexual ideology. Political liberalism takes the larger view that sexual ideologies are components of comprehensive doctrines, none of which, in a truly democratic society, rules the boundaries social life.

In the case of Restrictive sexual ideology where a morally virtuous life is attained by the adherence to moral absolutes and not through individually defined moral priorities, political liberalism's insistence on the exercise of reason under the conditions of freedom appears to refute Restrictive sexual ideology and place a stamp of approval on the ethics of Permissive sexual ideology. However, this conclusion misconstrues the nature of political liberalism. Political liberalism makes no judgements on the validity of believing in or living one's life according to the moral absolutes of Restrictive sexual ideology except in those cases where it extends itself into the realm of unreasonable doctrines. Indeed, political liberalism affirms the right of Restrictive sexual ideologues to express their views to their families, communities, and the public at large. Political liberalism is not interested in infringing on these rights. Political liberalism is interested only in affirming the right of others to arrive at and hold contrary views. It is only when Restrictive sexual ideology interferes with the right to consider alternative ideological perspectives that it runs afoul of political liberalism.

It is in this sense that the limited scope of political liberalism allows belief systems that appear to be in conflict with the free exercise of reason to persevere. In essence, this is because political liberalism does not recommend a specific or comprehensive view of the ends to which an individual's perception of the good life must lead. Although it often seems paradoxical, political liberalism allows individuals to adopt belief systems that rely on faith and obedience to authoritative rules rather than on liberal concepts of making individually deliberated free choices as a means of attaining the good life. Political liberalism demands only that the essential elements of the overlapping consensus of democratic society be respected in order to accommodate moral pluralism. Aside from this minimum, and presumably agreed upon, commitment to democratic values, individuals are free to think and behave as they wish. Moon (1993), articulates this basic aspect of political liberalism when he writes that

> Because political liberalism seeks to provide space for moral diversity, it does not offer a comprehensive view of the human good or a particular ideal of human excellence. In order to provide justifiable rules governing the public aspects of our lives, and to define the scope of liberty within which individuals can pursue their different visions,

> political liberalism must be committed to a limited, but widely shared, set of values and principles. These common values will be incomplete: a full moral life will necessarily have to incorporate other aims besides those of political liberalism. The common values will be based only on a "thin" conception of the self, one that abstracts a set of common elements from the contrasting views of the person held by different members of a society. (p. 9)

It is this "thin" conception of the self, the common values of the overlapping consensus, that is related to the higher order issues of political liberalism. A full moral life is reached through our individual appropriation of the lower order concepts of our respective sexual ideologies. In other words, lower order issues are part of what Rawls (1993) calls the background culture of the social world, whereas higher order issues involve the political culture and the fundamental values upon which it is based.

Thus, the exercise of reason under the conditions of freedom need not necessarily be seen as a disaster by the proponents of ideological perspectives that do not rely on reasoned deliberation in the process of doing sexual ethics. For political liberalism, the exercise of reason under the conditions of freedom does not apply to the internal workings of specific ethical systems. Rather, the exercise of reason under political liberalism refers only to the higher order opportunity for individuals to differentiate and choose between different ideological frameworks. Pluralism is respected when individuals exercise their reason to distinguish between and freely evaluate differing ideological perspectives. As Moon (1993) puts it, "political liberalism holds that democratic individuality is essential to create political community in the face of moral pluralism" (p. 99). Seeing the exercise of reason under the conditions of freedom as a disaster is strongly indicative of an ideological world view that is in conflict with the basic values of democracy as defined by political liberalism. It suggests an ideological perspective that is intolerant of moral pluralism.

Where sexual ideology does extend itself to the point of prescribing its particular vision as compulsory for all people, it is rejected by political liberalism. According to Moon (1993), in such a case, "one side claims a privileged access to truth and so refuses to engage in a search for ways of living together peacefully. Conflicts involving certain kinds of religious beliefs may be of this nature, and they are deeply troubling" (p. 9). Situations of this kind are what Moon (1993) calls the tragic conflicts of political liberalism.

On some issues, we may face tragic conflicts, conflicts in which all parties justify their positions in terms of what they regard as fundamental moral considerations, which are opposed in ways that do not permit reconciliation. Under such circumstances, political community must give way to imposition: whatever decision is taken, some will experience the outcome as unjust but will be constrained to abide by its terms. Moreover, and more significantly, the institutions and practices that political liberalism supports or even requires may unfairly burden some citizens, leading them to experience those norms as impositions. (p. 98)

Thus, it is possible that from some ideological perspectives, the exercise of freedom under the conditions of freedom, as I have described them, may be seen as offensive. Here, political liberalism does force an ideology into retreat, but only to the point where the ideology must reconcile itself to acknowledging, under the terms of the overlapping consensus, the right of opposing ideological perspectives to enter into public discourse.

With respect to sexuality, this problem is perhaps the most apparent with some religious perspectives toward sexual morality. However, it is also likely that the public expression of certain views related to sexuality will also be profoundly offensive to the proponents of some versions of Permissive sexual ideology. For example, it may be intolerable to some proponents of Permissive sexual ideology that we might entertain in public forums the notion that homosexuality is immoral or that traditional gender roles are beneficial. In some cases, political liberalism will place unappealing burdens on Permissive sexual ideology just as it will for Restrictive sexual ideology in other cases.

These unappealing burdens are necessary if we are to adequately and fairly address the fact that "In the contemporary world we face the often difficult—and sometimes tragic—tasks of living with moral pluralism and managing moral conflict" (Ibid., p. 35). The burden that acknowledging the right of opposing views to be expressed places on the proponents of various ideological perspectives is a constraint that is basic to the fundamentals of democracy. Such a constraint fairly regulates interactions between individuals and groups whose moral beliefs differ in significant ways.

Conclusion

As the history of sexuality shows, the affirmation of ideological pluralism—a respect by all parties for the overlapping consensus of democracy—has been, in the sexual arena, particularly hard to come by. As Weeks (1992) observes in an essay titled "Values in an Age of Uncertainty," "Many writers seem to want to give up the struggle altogether as they assert the impossibility of agreeing on values whatsoever" (p. 397). Weeks correctly points out that we need "to achieve a new style of debate about values" and that "sexual values are the supreme challenge of the recognition of difference" (p. 403). "Is it possible, then, to construct a common normative standard by which we can affirm different identities and ways of life? Can we balance relativism and some sense of minimal universal values?" (Ibid., p. 405).

In answer to this question, Weeks proposes that the supreme challenge of addressing sexual values in a society characterized by value conflict can be met through what he calls *radical pluralism*. In crucial respects, Weeks' radical pluralism is compatible with Rawls conception of political liberalism in that "radical pluralism draws on central values in the liberal tradition: its commitment to toleration and individual autonomy above all" (Weeks, p. 406). According to Weeks,

> the achievement of a radical and plural democracy is a project to be constructed, a set of values to be worked for against the institutional barriers that inhibit the possibilities of its realization. Radical pluralism is an argument for a more open and democratic culture which does not assume any historic inevitability nor any *a priori* justification in "the nature of human kind." (p. 407)

Whereas in a culture drawn from radical pluralism the individual and groups of persons bound together by common beliefs have the right to toleration and autonomy with respect to their sexual values, they are limited by their obligation to accord these same rights to others with contrary beliefs. Within such a culture, "many truths would flourish" (Weeks, 1992, p. 406). Weeks (1995) expands on this position somewhat by calling for "democratic autonomy" (p. 65) as a means of democratizing sexuality, enabling individuals "equal opportunities to pursue one's choices and life chances without blocking the equal rights of others" (p. 66). In other words,

> Democratic autonomy puts the obligation on the individual to express his or her desires in ways which respect the claims of the other in forms which are moral for that individual, and which acknowledge and attempt to deal with the inequalities which inevitably intrude between social actors. (Ibid.)

In these respects, Weeks' programme for sexual values appears compatible with the central goals of political liberalism. Given the importance of sexuality in shaping our culture, this approach to sexual values can play a significant role in creating and maintaining a democratic society.

Relying on Rawls' (1993) conception of political liberalism, I have outlined a basic philosophical framework for accommodating opposing sexual ideologies within the context of a democratic culture. It has been suggested that a plurality of reasonable yet incompatible sexual ideologies is the normal result of the democratic right of freedom of belief. A democratic culture assumes a collective acceptance of moral pluralism. In turn, a democratic culture assumes a collective acceptance of the existence and flourishing of a plurality of reasonable yet incompatible sexual ideologies.

Further, within the context of a democratic society, the existence of a plurality of sexual ideologies is to be tolerated and affirmed by the public institutions of a democratic regime. Specific sexual ideologies are to be tolerated and affirmed provided they are reasonable in that they remain faithful to the overlapping consensus of a democratic society. Here, being reasonable does not mean being logically consistent with a particular sexual ideology. Being reasonable means respecting the right of all people to freedom of belief. This implies that the proponents of specific sexual ideologies are to refrain from imposing their beliefs on others. Central to the theory of political liberalism is the contention that the overlapping consensus itself is not derived from a particular ideology, but is drawn from the basic moral principles affirmed by all people who willingly accept and affirm democratic living. This, in theory, contributes to the placing of divergent and opposing sexual ideologies on a level playing field.

In the search for a reasonable, fair, and coherent philosophy of sexuality education in the schools, political liberalism offers a theoretical framework for sexuality education that is consistent with the essential values of democracy. Given the highly divisive and ideologically laden nature of the debate around sexuality education in the schools, a broad base of at least reluctant support for a democratic philosophy of education may provide the best hope of providing our young people with a meaningful and effective sexuality education that is appropriate to a democratic society characterized by moral pluralism.

In most cases, a democratic philosophy of sexuality education implies a radical alteration of existing sexuality education practice. Most importantly, it encourages students to think about sexuality not simply in the context of their own ideological perspective or simply in the context of whatever happens to be the dominant ideological discourse of the day. Rather, it encourages students to think about sexuality within the context of democratic values. Just as importantly, a democratic sexuality education provides students with the opportunity to deliberate between different ideological perspectives in forming their own value positions related to sexuality. As Manley-Casimir and Sussel (1987) aptly put it, for rights-based democratic societies "...being able to make informed decisions between conflicting values forms a central feature of political socialization" (p. 172).

Note

1. In *Political Liberalism*, Rawls (1993) does not address the applications of this theory for sexuality. However, in *A Theory of Justice*, Rawls (1971) does, according to Ruse (1988, p. 248) remark "tangentially that the principles of justice do require the state to tolerate sexual relationships which some find degrading or shameful."

CHAPTER SIX

Sexuality Education: Towards Democracy

━━··━━━··━━━━··━━━··━━━··━━━··━━━··━━━··━━━··━━━··━━━··━━━··━

To date, the generally accepted view of education has been that young people should be challenged intellectually in school, that they should be taught to think critically, to solve problems, and to use their judgement and imagination. Concomitant to this is the belief that as these skills are developed, a respect for the opinions of others should be fostered.

(Spindel & Duby, 1994)

The primary goal of sexuality education should be substantially the same as that for education in all subjects, that is, to provide the individual, over the course of the K-12 school experience, with knowledge and thinking skills necessary to understanding self and society, and the relationship between the two, as well as skills to make positive contributions, however minute, to the shaping of this society and the course of its history....It is of great importance that students learn something of the values and world views which different groups have held historically and currently hold along with conflicts generated by opposing views. Sexuality education devoted to critical inquiry should strive to increase historical consciousness not contribute to historical amnesia.

(Pollis, 1985)

Introduction

The battle over sexuality in both the school and society has been shaped by the question of whether it is the values of Restrictive or Permissive sexual ideology that should be supported as the sexual ethics of our culture. To use Rawls' (1993) terms, this debate has not focussed on reaching an overlapping consensus consistent with the principles of political liberalism, but rather, as the debate is currently set up, it is focussed on seeing which comprehensive doctrine (sexual ideology) will emerge victorious. In other words, the goal of the debate is not a resolution that respects either democratic procedures or individual rights within a democracy. Rather, the goal for the debaters seems to be to establish social and political supremacy for their respective sexual ideology.

The ideological nature of the debate about sexuality education, in particular, is often masked by the tendency to deny that one's own views are ideologically based. It is noteworthy that when the proponents of particular approaches to sexuality education criticize their opponents, they typically do so by referring to the opposing point of view in terms of the ideology that it reflects. We are quick to label those who disagree with us as ideologues. The proponents of comprehensive sexuality education are sometimes accused of, for example, "ideologically pushing religious humanism via sex-ed" (Gardiner, 1992, p. 262) or it is suggested that "The unifying core of comprehensive sex education is not intellectual but ideological" (Dafoe-Whitehead, 1994, p. 70). The proponents of abstinence-only sexuality education are frequently described in terms of their adherence to a "fixed world view" (e.g., Yarber, 1992) or "far-right" (e.g., Sedway, 1992) ideology. I have tried to show that there is some credibility to the view that various perspectives on sexuality education are instrumentally informed by a larger sexual ideology. It is striking, however, that we rarely use the concept of ideology to refer to, and assess, our own point of view. This is because within the discourse on sexuality and sexuality education the concept of ideology is frequently employed as a rhetorical tool to denounce opposing points of view. In other words, a critical conception of ideology with a negative connotation is more likely to occur in this discourse than is a neutral conception of ideology which focusses on, in a less judgemental fashion, the normative structure of systems of belief.[1]

The tendency to employ a critical conception of ideology in the discourse on sexuality education is problematic in that it obscures how each of us, as a proponent of a particular point of view, approaches the debate on sexuality education. It is only those who are on the wrong side of the debate who hold ideologies. To hold an opinion derived from ideology is to hold an unworthy opinion. A critical conception of ideology inhibits us from seeing that we also, no matter from what point of view, consciously or unconsciously have an ideology of our own. Unless we are ready to engage in the necessary self-reflection to recognize and acknowledge the tenets of our own sexual ideologies, an overlapping consensus upon which a truly democratic sexuality education in the schools can be created will be out of reach. As Pollis, (1985) puts it, we need to find

> a vehicle for understanding why debates on the content and methods of sexuality education are frequently like ships passing in the night with participants talking past, rather than with, one another. What is put forward as a reasonably impartial, value-free analysis based on facts and theories is more or less burdened by value judgements flowing from a world view which remains unarticulated. (p. 285)

An analysis of these debates that contextualizes differing perspectives in terms of their sexual ideology may provide such a vehicle. Such an analysis, because it is concerned not with establishing the correctness of particular ideologies but rather with seeking to find points of convergence in the affirmation and respect for the core values of democracy, needs, as far as possible, to employ a neutral conception of ideology.

We can only hope to reach a workable solution to the debates about sexuality education when, at the larger social/political level, policy makers and the public at large see the debates not as a battle between good and evil, but as a discourse between two very different groupings of ideological thought, each with its own distinctive ethical perspective and each with a well-established presence in Western society. A philosophy of sexuality education derived from an overlapping consensus of reasonable, yet conflicting, sexual ideologies offers a framework for the form and content of sexuality education programs that accommodate moral pluralism. This overlapping consensus is to be abstracted from that limited or "thin" set of values that we presumably all share by virtue of our collective endorsement of the right to freedom of belief, conscience, religion, etc.

This does not mean that the fundamentalist Christian needs to give up her belief that homosexuality is morally wrong and against the laws of nature, any more than it means that the secular psychologist needs to give up his belief that gays, lesbians, and bisexuals are as psychologically healthy as heterosexuals. The Jehovanist still believes in God and The Naturalist still believes in science. The Romanticist still believes that no teenager should have sex and the Libertarian still believes that it is permissable if it is consenting and protected. Commitment to the overlapping consensus of democracy as a guide for educating youth about sexuality does not mean the sacrificing of one's own beliefs. It also does not mean that we must share our opponents beliefs, particularly as they pertain to moral issues, but simply that we accord them the opportunity for expression within the context of a democratic culture and that this occurs also in education.

Some people lament the fact that we live in a time where our culture is not possessed by a single rigid vision of the truth. However, the absence of a consensus on an absolute truth perhaps pushes us to embrace the core values of democracy: the right to believe what we believe, to live, within reasonable limits, as we wish to live, and to respect the right of others to do the same in an equal and autonomous fashion. In political terms, this means that

> our exercise of political power is fully proper only when it is exercised in accordance with a constitution the essentials of which all citizens as free and equal may reasonably be expected to endorse in light of the principles and ideals acceptable to their common human reason. (Rawls, 1993, p. 137)

In a democracy these principles and ideals are expressed through the values of "equal political and civil liberty; fair equality of opportunity; the values of economic reciprocity; the social bases of mutual respect between citizens" (Ibid., p. 139).

To the extent that we, as a democratic society, share a commitment to these values, not everything is subjective. We have a free-standing view, a kind of objectivity if you will, that provides a basis for social life, including sexual life as it pertains to these freedoms and responsibilities. This is the overlapping consensus of democratic societies "without which political liberalism would merely be a doctrine, not a conception providing for political legitimacy and stability" (Hoffman, 1995, p. 54).

The great advantage of living in an age of uncertainty is that it can be highly conducive to a democratic political, intellectual, and social climate. The admission, or even affirmation, of a lack of a collective consensus or certainty makes the encouragement of freedom of belief more tenable. The totalitarian is often characterized by his utter certainty that he knows the truth or that he is certain that objective truth does not exist. If I am certain that I have a grasp on matters of truth, I may have less hesitancy to impose my beliefs on others. After all, I am introducing them, albeit coercively, to the way things really are or should be. When armed with absolute certainty, one may have the tendency to favour "education in the right values." As Haydon (1995) suggests,

> This is a view, of course, that can only be put into practice by those who believe they know what the right values are. This means already

that the authoritative answer view faces difficulties in a context of moral pluralism. Not only is there not unanimity on what the right values are, but there is disagreement on what it means to call certain values the right ones, and on what kind of enquiry—philosophical, theological, or even anthropological or biological—is relevant to establishing any such claim. (p. 56)

The embracing of one truth, one ideology, is often the gist of sexuality education in our public schools. Indeed, it is fair to say that sexuality education is often ruled by a comprehensive doctrine rather than by an overlapping consensus of limited but shared values. In this respect, it may be argued, with considerable justification, that much of contemporary sexuality education in the public schools is profoundly undemocratic.

The undemocratic nature of contemporary sexuality education has a number of disturbing implications. Sexuality education programs tainted by ideological dominance or controversy are unable to fulfil young people's inalienable right to freedom of belief and the opportunity to critically deliberate between competing ideological perspectives. In the face of our continuing ideological strife around sexuality, such programs also do little to contribute to a democratic social/political culture. Finally, sexuality education programs that replace the critical exploration of sexual ideology with the promotion of one particular ideological perspective are less likely to help students who do not share that perspective to protect their own sexual health.

The Meaning of Democratic Education

Theodore Kaltsounis (1994) writes that "social studies, as a subject in the school curriculum, lacks a solid foundation, and is therefore in a state of crisis" (p. 176). Kaltsounis (1994) also observes that attempts to state a clear purpose for social studies have either been ineffective or "At their worst, they reflect the philosophical or ideological biases of those advancing some particular solution" (p. 176). Sexuality education, which might well be considered a type of social studies, suffers from a similar malaise.

Although it is certainly fertile ground for philosophical discourse, academic philosophers of education have largely avoided the subject of sexuality education (Diorio, 1982). Aside from highly generalized statements regarding sexual health, few sexuality education curricula contain clear philosophical statements offering a rationale for the program's content

(LaCursia, Beyer, & Ogletree, 1994). And, as I have tried to show, sexuality education has been guided more often than not by ideological bias rather than a solid philosophical foundation.

Kaltsounis (1994) offers a solution for the philosophical crisis afflicting social studies.

> American social studies educators do not need to look far for a strong foundation. They have only to stop taking democracy for granted and make its content, principles, practices, and history the main source, inspiration, and substance of social studies....Everything in the program should actively advance understanding of democracy and the values and behaviors associated with it. American schools must stop doing things in social studies because of habit or tradition, and must provide America's youth instead with a truly democratic citizenship education. (p. 180)

Mosher, Kenny, and Garrod (1994) argue that education modelled on democratic principles is important because, among other things,

> (1) democracy is vitally dependant on a responsive, educated citizenry; (2) children educated in democratic groups benefit personally as well as in terms of social development; (3) democratic participation contributes to the growth of minds; and (4) democracy has to be recreated in the understanding and behavior of each new generation of citizens or it is jeopardized. (p. 24)

Philosophers of education interested in how the educational process can contribute to democracy on both an individual and societal level have emphasized the necessity for individuals to acquire the ability to deliberate critically between competing points of view (e.g., Guttman, 1987; Weinstein, 1991). This enables them, as individuals, not only to freely choose between competing conceptions of the good life but also to participate in society as democratic citizens. In other words, the principle that education, if it is to be considered truly democratic, must facilitate the ability to critically deliberate between competing conceptions of the good life is important for two reasons. First, it contributes to the individual's democratic right to freely choose a conception of the good life. Secondly, it contributes to the conscious social reproduction of democratic values and thus helps to create or maintain the democratic nature of society. As Amy Guttman (1987) puts it her book *Democratic Education*, it would be an illegitimate pretension to educational authority on anyone's part to deprive any child of the capacities necessary for choice among good lives. The pretension would be illegitimate for two reasons. First: even if I know that my way of life is best, I cannot transform this claim into the claim that I have a right to impose my way of life on anyone else, even on my own child, at the cost of depriving her of the capacity to choose a good life. Second: many if not all of the capacities necessary for choice among good lives are also necessary for choice among good societies. A necessary (but not sufficient) condition of conscious social reproduction is that citizens have the capacity to deliberate among alternative ways of personal and political life. To put this point in more liberal language: a good life and a good society for self-reflective people require (respectively) individual and collective freedom of choice. (p. 40)

Mark Cladis (1995), in an essay examining the sociologist/philosopher Emile Durkheim's thoughts on the relationship between education and democracy, suggests that "Through moral education, youth become autonomous and develop the skills in reflective and critical thought that are so important to flourishing democracies, as they are nurtured in society's shared 'ideas, sentiments, and practices'" (p. 37). In sum, democratic moral education promotes autonomy and critical thought within the context of the shared beliefs and practices of society.

As we have seen, autonomy as conceived by political liberalism, entails that people think of themselves as free in that they are able to independently form a self-authenticating conception of the good life. In other words, the individual is free from either explicit or implicit bias or coercion in forming value positions. However, arriving at a genuinely autonomous conception of the good life requires the ability to think critically. Autonomous judgement is the end product of the critical thinking process.

Indeed, the ability to think critically can justifiably be seen as the single most essential ingredient of moral education appropriate for a plural democracy characterized by divergent moral perspectives. This is because critical thinking gives us "the ability to make rational judgements relevant to political life, and thus, can be seen as essential for the preparation of citizens in a democracy" (Weinstein, 1991, p. 9). Critical thinking enables us to freely and rationally differentiate, evaluate, and choose between competing conceptions of the good life. "The purpose of critical deliberation is to maximize the possibility of reconsidering what constitutes good lives and good societies by maximizing the available alternatives" (Weinstein, 1991, p. 11). Critical thinking helps students intellectually process different points of view, particularly in regard to socially and politically sensitive issues.

In a society which affirms democratic pluralism,

> there is a need for education, not just in morals, but about morality: an education that will give people some knowledge and understanding not just of a variety of moral positions in the world, but of various ways in which moral values enter into people's lives and some knowledge, too, of the kinds of arguments that have been used to support moral positions and, unavoidably, of the existence of various sorts of scepticism about morals. (Haydon, 1995, pp. 62-63)

A democratic education clearly must try to create conditions amenable to autonomy and critical deliberation. However, although their presence is necessary, in and of themselves, autonomy and critical deliberation are insufficient for addressing the moral implications of learning to live in a democratic society. In order to be fully democratic in its function, education must help people reflect upon their rights and responsibilities as they relate to the overlapping consensus of a pluralistic democracy. This constitutes a very limited, but highly substantive, claim about the nature and purpose of moral discourse within a democratic education.

This is a limited claim because it has little or nothing to say about the real or precise nature of morality itself. Consequently, a democratic education avoids teaching students to accept any one vision of the nature of morality. To make such an attempt would involve invoking a comprehensive doctrine as the preferred philosophical basis for understanding morality. So, for example, introducing into the classroom moral theories drawn from theism or atheism as the most valid or only acceptable way of doing ethics violates the overlapping consensus of democracy by imposing a comprehensive doctrine. As Haydon (1995) suggests in his discussion of the implications of democratic pluralism for moral education, "both theism and atheism would be parts of different comprehensive doctrines; political liberalism is not part of comprehensive doctrine, but is that set of principles, of an explicitly political sort, on which different comprehensive views can converge" (p. 55).

Although minimalist in its framework for moral discourse, addressing moral issues in a democratic education can be an intellectually challenging

endeavour, purposefully directed at learning, among other things, to nego-
tiate different moral perspectives within the context of the assigned rights
and responsibilities of democratic citizenship. This is the substantive moral
element of a democratic sexuality ducation.

In order for students to engage in this process of democratic moral
reflection, they must acquire a reasonably thorough understanding of differing sexual ideologies including the world views that support them. This
kind of understanding is important because ideological perspectives "color
the way in which each of us approaches a particular political, economic, or
moral issue, as well as the way we reach decisions about sexual issues and
relationships" (Francoeur, 1989, p. xix). It requires an understanding by
students of their own moral perspective as well as those of their peers, family,
religion, and community. Most importantly, bringing a substantive moral
element to a democratic sexuality education requires the examination of
one's own personal sexual ideology, its history, its sources of moral knowledge and wisdom, and its behavioural norms in relation to the values that
make up the overlapping consensus of democratic society.

This type of sexuality education, however, is bound to be disconcerting
to many people. Encouraging students to critically deliberate between
competing points of view in sexuality education is something that is more
than likely to be greeted with considerable opposition. For example, parents
who hold a particular sexual ideology and have raised their children to follow
that same ideology may well be highly uncomfortable with the idea of having
their children exposed to alternative value positions. As Haydon (1995)
suggests,

> Parents who have tried their best to instil in their children the values
> which they believe to be right may reasonably be suspicious that an
> education that gives their children knowledge of different values held
> by others, and teaches their children to reflect critically on these
> values, may only succeed only in unravelling the good work that they
> have done. (p. 54)

From the standpoint of a democratic philosophy of education two points
need to be made in regard to this concern. First, young people need, in order
to become truly democratic citizens, a knowledge and understanding of
moral perspectives that differ from their own familial, religious, ethnic, and
social traditions. Because democracy requires a basic minimal respect and
toleration between peoples holding different moral doctrines, an equitably

organized peaceful co-existence of diverse perspectives in society requires some understanding of beliefs that differ from one's own. As Cladis (1995) notes,

> Future citizens of democracies need to know about styles of belief and practices other than that of their family or local group. Otherwise a child, a future adult who had been held captive to a highly particular moral point of view, could find it difficult to respect those holding other worthy views. (p. 40)

A second, and equally important, point in regard to this question relates to the manner and conviction with which we hold our values. It is often assumed by the proponents of both Restrictive and Permissive sexual ideology that the mere exposure to "offensive" sexual values will weaken young people's belief in the "right" values which may have already been communicated to youth by parents or other authoritative sources. A democratic sexuality education, therefore, according to this view, becomes a corrupting force.

From the standpoint of a democratic philosophy of education, this view reflects a misunderstanding of the dynamics in which citizens in a democracy are invited to form their beliefs. As Haydon (1995) puts it, "Genuine attachment to a particular set of values does not come through uncontested blind acceptance but rather through the critical appropriation of those values when rigorously compared to alternative value systems" (p. 61). In other words, genuine attachment to the lower order set of values specific to a particular sexual ideology is less likely to occur through explicit, unadulterated imposition, but more likely to occur through a positive evaluation of that ideology in comparison to others. Compared to the direct inculcation of particular beliefs, the opportunity for critical deliberation between differing points of view better enables people to fully understand, articulate, and defend their own views. According to Kelly (1986), strict partisans of a particular point of view who employ the educational methods of exclusive partiality,

> preclude the opportunity for realizing an informed and defensible position. Hence, by failing to expose students to the best alternative arguments and how presumably these can be effectively rebutted, the strict partisan is essentially fabricating intellectual straw people vulnerable to the serious challenges from competent adversaries. In a tightly closed society where conflicting perspectives are suppressed or

nonexistent, the strict partisan's approach to preserving allegiance is perhaps feasible. In a more pluralistic culture, however, a cocooned existence is constantly in jeopardy; as a result, the presumption that individuals can be protected from multiple influences is dubious, if not myopic. More likely, the fragile proteges of the strict partisan face any of several ominous futures: defensive dogmatism, disillusionment and paralysis, ethical relativism, or defection to the enemy camp. While the most appealing of these, dogmatism, may look and feel familiar to the strict partisan, it is an improbable strategy for durably seducing or converting an inquiring mind. (p. 119)

In sum, for strict partisans of both Restrictive and Permissive sexual ideology, the educational methods of exclusive partiality have a strong potential for self-defeating failure. Recipients of exclusively partial sexuality education have a greater vulnerability to confusion in a society characterized by a plurality of often conflicting sexual value systems. In addition, they may be more likely to reject the value system that they have uncritically inherited from their familial, ethnic, religious tradition or from their formal education. As difficult as it may be for true believers in particular sexual ideologies to fathom, their respective ideological interests may be best served by advocating for an education that exposes young people not only to the best arguments of the true believers' ideology but also to the best arguments of contrary points of view. If the true believer's ideology is defensible when subject to rigorous critical deliberation, as few true believer's would deny, then an education that provides the opportunity for such deliberation should be encouraged and not rejected.

Striking a balance between a public education system founded on the politically secular principles of democratic education and the interests of religious traditions has been highly precarious. It is a particularly contentious issue when viewed in the context of sexuality education. It is a commonly made complaint that sexuality education which fails to inculcate religious values constitutes an assault on those values. It is argued that sexuality education becomes a platform for indoctrinating students into an acceptance of secular sexual morality. The rejoinder by defenders of comprehensive sexuality education that their programs promote "universal human values" has been insufficient to quell the concerns of Restrictive sexual ideologues.

This type of dispute is born as much out of a misunderstanding of the nature of education appropriate for democratic societies as it is out of a genuinely rational conflict of perspective. Here, the doctrine of comprehensive liberalism—a comprehensive doctrine like any other—which is generally compatible with some major strands of Permissive sexual ideology is mistaken for political liberalism which is the basic underpinning of a democratic philosophy of education. Ideally, a democratic education neither subverts religious values nor promotes secular ones. But it does educate young people in the values that must be respected as requirements of democratic citizenship. The fact that these values, although not antagonistic to reasonable religious doctrines, are primarily secular in their justification can indicate a bias, in the view of some defenders of a religiously based education, in the direction of secularism. Rawls (1993) notes this problem when he writes that

> Here it may be objected that requiring children to understand the political conception in these ways is in effect, though not in intention, to educate them to a comprehensive liberal conception. Doing the one may lead to the other, if only because once we know the one, we may of our own accord go on to the other. It must be granted that this may indeed happen in the case of some. And certainly there is some resemblance between the values of political liberalism and the values of the comprehensive liberalisms of Kant and Mill. But the only way this objection can be answered is to set out carefully the great differences in both scope and generality between political and comprehensive liberalism. (pp. 199-200)

In responding to this concern, a clear distinction must be made between a sexuality education derived from political liberalism and a sexuality education derived from comprehensive liberalism. Sexuality education derived from comprehensive liberalism is likely to resemble many existing forms of permissive sexuality education. In other words, it employs the lower order moral precepts of Permissive sexual ideology, often based on secular liberal philosophy, as the over-riding philosophical context for addressing sexual issues in the classroom. In contrast, a sexuality education derived from political liberalism is based on the higher order principle of accommodating a diversity of lower order ideological perspectives. This suggests that neither particular religious nor secular liberal conceptions of sexual ethics are accorded a privileged position. Indeed, this principle is at the very heart of democracy in general and of a democratic philosophy of sexuality education. Within such an education any reasonable doctrine is afforded an equal opportunity, through critical deliberation, to be appropriated by those students who see virtue in it.

Thus, it is the case that a democratic sexuality education encourages students to choose their own sexual ideology within the overlapping consensus of the higher order values of freedom of belief and critical deliberation. It would be a mistake, however, to assume that within the confines of a democratic society, education of this kind is biased against Restrictive sexual ideology and in favour of Permissive ideology. This assumption only holds true if sexuality education programs take their cue from the lower order precepts of Permissive sexual ideology. In such a case, sexuality education would rightly be seen as undemocratic. However, to assume that democratic sexuality education, a form of sexuality education that does not directly inculcate Restrictive sexual ideology is, by its very nature, necessarily and unfairly biased against Restrictive sexual ideology, is to assume that the principles of freedom of belief and critical deliberation must also be incompatible with Restrictive sexual ideology. Where it is the case that one maintains this assumption, one is forced either to argue against democratic education or to recognize that the assumed incompatibility between democratic sexuality education and Restrictive sexual ideology represents what Moon (1993) calls a tragic conflict of political liberalism. In the latter circumstance, the Restrictive sexual ideologue who holds this assumption must accept, if he or she is to remain faithful to the overlapping consensus in support of freedom of belief, what he or she will perceive as an unreasonable burden.

In sum, the participants in the discourse on sexuality education, whether they be parents, teachers, or policy makers, need to keep in mind the distinction between the relative and appropriate roles of both religious and secular interpretations of sexual morality and the overarching higher order structures of political liberalism when putting forth proposals for the form and content of sexuality education.

If it can be agreed that the guiding principles of democracy and democratic education, as I have articulated them here, should replace sexual ideology as the guiding force behind sexuality education in the schools, then a broad picture of a democratic philosophy of sexuality education begins to emerge.

First, a democratic philosophy of sexuality education begins not with truth statements about the nature of human sexuality, but with a commitment to promote the values of democracy. Indeed, because issues related to sexuality such as homosexuality, gender relations, and teen sexuality are among the most significant and divisive social issues of our time, sexuality education may be the ideal forum for young people to contemplate the meaning and implications of democratic principles for the way in which our society addresses sexuality.

Secondly, a democratic philosophy of sexuality education does not suggest that there is a single moral ideal of human sexual conduct. Rather, a democratic philosophy of sexuality education acknowledges and affirms the existence of a diversity of sexual moral truths. Students need to acquire a basic knowledge and understanding of the various ideological perspectives toward sexuality in our culture.

Thirdly, in addressing student's own personal beliefs about sexuality, a democratic philosophy of sexuality education provides the opportunity for students to recognize and reflect upon their own values and those of their peers, families, communities, and society at large. This approach is essential if young people are to be accorded their inalienable right to freedom of belief, conscience, religion, etc.

Fourthly, in addressing the social aspects of human sexuality, students are encouraged to reflect upon their own values and those of others in the context of the overlapping consensus of a democratic society. This constitutes the most explicitly moral component of the process of sexuality education. It makes clear the sexual rights and responsibilities of individuals in a democratic society. It invites reflection by students on the degree to which different beliefs may or may not be compatible with the overlapping consensus of common democratic values.

Fifthly, in teaching the information and skills to prevent unwanted pregnancy and infection with HIV and other sexually transmitted diseases, a democratic philosophy of sexuality education stipulates that such education fully respects the needs and values of all students. In other words, a democratic sexuality education must, if it is to remain democratic, teach the information and skills to avoid sexual activity in order to respect the needs and values of those students who choose to be abstinent and it must also teach the information and skills to practise safer sex in order to respect the needs and values of those students who choose to be sexually active.

The recently published *Canadian Guidelines for Sexual Health Education* (Health Canada, 1994) offer a representative example of a democratic philosophy of sexuality education. This document represents one of the few cases in the Western world where a national government has issued guidelines for sexuality education. Because Canada is generally held by its citizens and government to be a pluralistic and democratic state, the working group mandated to create the guidelines were committed to an approach to sexuality education that accommodates moral pluralism. In other words, the Canadian guidelines "were formulated to embody an educational philosophy that is inclusive, respects diversity, and reflects the fundamental precepts of education in a democratic society" (McKay & Barrett, 1995, p. 65).

Among the introductory statements to the guidelines is the following:

> The terms "sexual health" and "sexual health education" mean different things to different people, depending on their experiences, values and customs. This document recognizes and welcomes such diversity. In spite of such diversity, however, there are common principles, aspirations and expectations upon which to build national Canadian Guidelines for Sexual Health Education. (Health Canada, 1994, p. 4)

This statement makes two points supportive of a democratic philosophy of sexuality education. First, it acknowledges that sexuality has different meanings for different people, suggesting a recognition of the divergent sexual ideologies that exist in Canada. Further, the guidelines suggest that "Sexual health educators should remain open to the range of meanings and understandings associated with the term 'sexual health'" (Ibid., p. 29). Secondly, the above statement refers to "common principles, aspirations, and expectations," to guide sexuality education, suggesting that there are common values that can be abstracted, with respect to human sexuality, from the diverse background culture of Canadian society.

Of the ten philosophy statements that accompany the guidelines, three are particularly salient in their compatibility with a democratic philosophy of sexuality education. "Effective sexual health education enhances sexual health within the context of an individual's values, moral beliefs, religious or ethno-cultural background, sexual orientation or other such characteristic" (Ibid., p. 8). This statement acknowledges and affirms that individuals are to have their values respected in the delivery of sexuality education, supporting the democratic principle of freedom of belief. The guidelines further support this principle through the statement that "Effective sexual health education is structured so that attitudinal and behavioural changes arise out of informed individual choice and are not imposed by an external authority" (Ibid.).

These statements in support of freedom of belief are balanced by another statement which states that, "In addition, effective sexual health education provides, within the domain of its subject matter, accurate information that counters misunderstanding and reduces discrimination based upon race, gender, sexual orientation, religion, ethnocultural background or disability" (Ibid.). This statement can be reasonably interpreted as functioning, within the context of sexuality education, as a remedy to one of the key dilemmas of liberal democratic cultures. In this particular case, the guidelines identify the principle of nondiscrimination to mediate a clash of beliefs and rights where one set of beliefs comes into direct conflict with another set of beliefs. The principle of nondiscrimination is introduced to challenge beliefs that, when put into practice, infringe on the rights of others. In this case, beliefs supporting discriminatory acts constitute an unreasonable doctrine, falling outside the boundaries of the overlapping consensus. Although the guidelines support the principles consistent with the freedoms inherent in a politically liberal culture that sexuality education should take place within the context of an individual's moral beliefs and that attitudes and behaviour arise out of informed individual choice, these freedoms are limited by the principle of nondiscrimination. If the principle of nondiscrimination is held to be part of the overlapping consensus of basic values abstracted from the common culture, the balancing of freedoms in this approach to sexuality education is consistent with the theory of political liberalism.

Conclusion: Implications for Teaching and Learning

Sexuality education is perhaps unique among the topics included in the contemporary school curriculum in that students, particularly teenagers, are almost universally receptive to learning more about human sexuality. Rarely do we meet an adolescent who does not have an unquenchable thirst for sexual knowledge. Thus, I was not surprised to find, in my own research, that over 88% of adolescents between the age of 12 and 18 that I surveyed agreed with the statement "It is important for teenagers to receive sexual health education" (McKay & Holowaty, 1997). In other words, compared to some other school topics, sexuality educators should have little problem getting the attention of their charges. However, young people's interest in sexuality does not mean that sophistocated discussions of sexual morality in the context of democratic values is an appropriate starting point for a child's learning about sexuality. A democratic sexuality education proceeds and takes shape according to the developmental needs and capacities of the child and adolescent.

With respect to sexuality, children and very young adolescents tend to be grounded in highly practical, concrete issues: "How does pregnancy happen?"; "What does orgasm mean?"; "How do people get AIDS?"; "What's a homosexual?" In cognitive terms, the concrete operational child is seeking empirical reality. She is looking for concrete answers to concrete questions. Such children are not yet able to manipulate or fully comprehend abstract ideas. Children at this developmental level are likely to have considerable difficulty juxtaposing or reconciling different ideological perspectives on sexuality. The realm of ideology is of little interest and often beyond the cognitive capacity of the child entrenched in concrete operational thought. As developmental psychologist John Flavel (1985) aptly puts it, "A theorist the elementary school child is not" (p. 98).

Thus, childhood sexuality education need not be aimed, as a specific objective, toward actively engaging young children in abstract reflections related to differing ideological perspectives on sexuality and how they impact on the self and society. In many respects, age and developmentally appropriate sexuality education for children is relatively uncomplicated. Sexual anatomy and the physiology of reproduction can easily be taught in a manner that does not require immediate reference to ideology.

Teachers of younger children must very careful, however, not to let ideological influence taint their teaching of even the most basic aspects of sexuality. For example, many young children want to know why a man and a women would ever want to have sex. For many young children the whole idea sounds both silly and gross. The standard reply to such a query is often that men and women have sex in order to produce babies and sometimes it is added that sex is a way for men and women to express love for each other. Such an explanation appears innocuous enough at first glance, but upon further examination, left as it is, this standard way of explaining to young children why people have sex is heavily laden with sexual ideology. To teach young children that the only reasons people have sex is to produce babies and solidify loving relationships is to inculcate the values of Restrictive sexual ideology. Notice that the above explanation makes no mention of sexual desire or pleasure as reasons why people have sex. It is interesting to note that the diagrams used to teach children sexual anatomy often do not include the clitoris. Why? Because, it is thought that the clitoris has no reproductive function. Our heritage of Restrictive sexual ideology has often led us to deny to children the existence of the erotic dimensions of human sexuality. Notice also that the reproductive explanation denies the existence of homosexual desire. Although young children cannot be expected to critically debate what the proper purpose of human sexual behaviour is, this does not mean that educators cannot be comprehensive in their explanations of human sexuality, teaching a range of perspectives.

The emergence of puberty is a critical period for the development of the young person and also for the way we teach about sexuality. Not only is the adolescent body saying, sometimes with considerable urgency, that it is ready and willing to be sexual, but the type of questions and concerns that the adolescent has are no longer limited simply to issues of a concrete nature. "Am I gay/lesbian and what will it mean for my life if I am?" "I want to have sex but I'm not sure I'm ready." "Is it okay to have sex when you're not in love?" "How can I get my boyfriend to treat me better?" Here, the questions have moved from the concrete empirical to the more fluid and challenging sphere of the uncertain and the possible. These adolescents have entered the world of personal, family, and societal values, social perspective taking and morality. They have, in other words, landed, sometimes with a thud, on the mine field of Western culture's ambivalent, conflicting, and confusing thicket of sexual ideology.

As the maturation process brings on the physiological changes of puberty it also lays the foundation for the transformation of the individual's mental capacities from concrete operational thought to formal operational thought. This transformation in cognitive development has two crucial implications for adolescent sexuality and the potential success of a democratic sexuality education. First, inherent in the developmental process is the acquisition of social cognition. This is "cognition about people and what they do and ought to do. It includes thinking and knowledge about the self and others as individuals, about social relations between people, about social customs, groups, and institutions" (Flavel, 1985, p. 159). Secondly, "with the onset of formal operational thinking and the prospect of advancing to higher levels of moral reasoning, cognitive and moral judgement-making processes allow adolescents to consider the consequences of their own and others' sexual decisions" (Downs & Scarborough Hillje, 1993, p. 25). A clear marker of a democratic sexuality education is that within the domain of its subject matter, it seeks to contribute to rather than stifle the social and cognitive development of adolescents.

As the maturation process opens up the possibility for advances in cognitive development, teaching adolescents to deliberate critically between divergent ideological perspectives on sexuality not only facilitates the ability of students to improve their reasoning abilities but also as part of this advancement, empowered them with the skills to become democratic citizens. As the ability for social cognition develops there comes a point in a person's life where it becomes possible to recognize that one's sexuality and one's decisions and judgements about sexuality are not entirely a function of the self, but rather are embedded in a social/political framework that steers our course and impacts on our lives. It is only when we have developed an awareness of how the social environment impacts upon us that we can start to take meaningful steps to consciously interact with the environment in ways that promote our own self-defined interests and goals. Otherwise we are left effectively powerless, subject to the whims of the culture around us. In terms of sexuality, this can be perilous. Sexuality education that attempts to impose ideology as opposed to promoting critical thought is developmentally harmful in that it stunts the potential for social cognitive growth. This may partially explain why it is frequently observed that adolescents often appear not to be well equipped to make reasoned decisions about sexuality. All too frequently, our culture, including our schools, have sought to issue commandments about sexuality to adolescents rather than to assist them in developing the critical skills to make well thought out decisions.

The implications of a democratic sexuality education for teaching and learning are clear. Programs should proceed according to the developmental stages of children and adolescents. In particular, beginning in adolescence, sexuality education programs need to teach students to identify prevailing ideological positions on sexuality and what they suggest about what it means to live the good life. Students need to familiarize themselves with the modes of decision making employed by these ideologies and teachers need to help students apply critical thinking skills to compare and evaluate them. Most importantly, through this process teachers can help students discover and clarify which ideological perspectives are most appropriate as guides to making decisions about their own lives. This type of education is fully consistent with the principles of democratic living.

Because sexuality education is often burdened by ideological influences, it rarely meets the conditions of a democratic philosophy of education. When programs are dominated by either Restrictive or Permissive sexual ideology, the resulting approach of exclusive partiality clearly impinges on the right of individuals to freely choose a conception of the good life. In addition, programs that exclude any controversial material through an approach of exclusive neutrality fail to address sexuality in any meaningful way and therefore curtail the opportunity to critically appropriate sexual ideology.

Furthermore, and perhaps most importantly, programs that address moral issues related to sexuality by promoting a particular sexual ideology, or by saying nothing at all via exclusive neutrality, fail to prepare students for democratic citizenship. As I have suggested, facilitating the ability to deliberate between divergent points of view is a fundamental component of political socialization in a plural democracy. When one sexual ideology is put on a superior footing in relation to others, not only is critical deliberation shut down, but also, in a fairly direct way, understanding and respect for differing ideological conceptions is undermined. In sum, instead of critical deliberation and an exploration of how different beliefs about social practices related to sexuality can be adjudicated by democratic values, we are left only with indoctrination. Such an approach does little in terms of the intellectual, moral, or social development of individual students.

Note

1.   I refer the reader back to Chapter Two for a more complete distinction between a critical and neutral conception of ideology.

CHAPTER SEVEN

A Democratic Approach to Key Issues in Sexuality Education: Sexual Orientation, Gender Equality, and Unwanted Pregnancy/STD Prevention

> The handling of sex education represents a major philosophical inconsistency in American society: the belief that the social good is best achieved by enforcing ignorance of possible options rather than by informed choice.
>
> (Bateson & Goldsby, 1988)

Introduction

It is not my intention here to map out in detail what a democratic sexuality education looks like from beginning to end. Nearly every topic area in sexuality education is shrouded in controversy. My focus has been to articulate the basic philosophical parameters of a democratic sexuality education. However, the implications of a democratic philosophy of sexuality education for classroom practice can be made clearer by explicating, in some detail, how several of the most controversial subject areas in sexuality education can be conceptualized in the context of a democratic sexuality education. The subjects of sexual orientation, gender equality, and pregnancy/STD prevention are perhaps the most controversial. Thus, these are the three subject areas I will address in more detail.

The discussion of these issues in the classroom will inevitably be shaped, to a considerable extent, by the social and historical context in which these discussions take place. This is readily seen in the differences in the ways contemporary Western culture addresses the issues of sexual orientation and gender equality. Both issues are important indicators of the way in which the imposition of sexual ideology impedes democratic living. As Susan Moller Okin (1997) puts it,

> These are two of the many dimensions along which persons in our society are not afforded equal treatment—in which their different bodies or desires are made to affect considerably the ways in which and the extent to which they are able to be effective citizens and to lead personally fulfilling lives. (p. 44)

However, although they share many similarities, the current debates on the rights of homosexuals and women hinge on somewhat different questions. For example, while it has not always been the case, the issue of whether women are entitled to full equality with men is largely moot in contemporary Western discourse. While there is a wide array of contemporary perspectives on gender equality, the view that women should not, in principle, enjoy the same basic rights as men has been largely rejected by Western society. For this issue, it is not so much a question of whether or not gender inequality exists. The feminist movement has generally convinced us, as a society, that it does. Rather, the question now seems to be how genuine and appropriate forms of gender equality can be achieved. For example, what, if any, changes in gender related sexual scripts are required to bring about sexual equality between men and women?

With respect to sexual orientation, the social and political discourse in contemporary Western culture hinges on somewhat different questions in the sense that, compared to the general level of acceptance of the principle of equality as it applies to women, acceptance of the principle of equality as it applies to the rights of homosexuals is not so widely shared. Although there is certainly important discourse and debate occuring around the issue of what steps can be taken by our society to ensure the equal rights of gays, lesbians, and bisexuals, our current cultural discourse on sexual orientation has not progressed to the same degree as the discourse around gender equality. Therefore, in its current historical context, a democratic sexuality education will place emphasis on different aspects of these issues.

Addressing the Issue of Sexual Orientation

Homosexuality[1] is, without doubt, among the most divisive social issues confronting Western culture today. There is no other issue which so clearly divides Restrictive and Permissive sexual ideology. What issues related to sexual orientation should be taught in the schools and how they should be taught are perhaps the most volatile of the debates surrounding sexuality education. Homosexuality is, perhaps, *the* litmus test for how our society approaches sexuality, particularly in terms of the degree of diversity that we will tolerate. The debate over homosexuality is highly complex and, I believe, its appropriate parameters are commonly misunderstood. I will, therefore, devote considerable space to addressing the following questions: How should the issue of homosexuality be dealt with in a democratic society? Subsequently, how should it be dealt with within a democratic sexuality education? Answering questions of this sort requires, as Michael Ruse (1988) points out in *Homosexuality: A Philosophical Inquiry*, "an investigation into values; an ethical inquiry" (p. 236). In this exploration, we are asking basic questions about how society *ought* to address a specific aspect of identity and sexual expression. Inherent in these questions is the issue of how the basic rights and freedoms of democracy apply to the moral disagreements within our society about sexual orientation. And, although these questions immediately raise moral issues, it is specifically in the moral domain that the debate over homosexuality has run amok.

If we think that the solution for the social debate over homosexuality has, as its focus, the question of whether or not homosexual behaviour is immoral or not, we are asking the wrong question. Such a question is relevant to the world of sexual ideology but not necessarily to the world of political and social democracy. We cannot answer the question of the moral validity of homosexual behaviour without an appeal to sexual ideology. In a liberal democracy characterized by the existence and affirmation of ideological diversity, no amount of moral debate will lead us toward a resolution of issues such as the moral validity of homosexuality. In such a circumstance we must turn to the principles of democracy to mediate between conflicting ideologies. Thus, we must, from a social policy perspective, examine homosexuality as a higher order issue of sexual morality. An approach to the issue of homosexuality that is consistent with the fundamental precepts of democracy, and therefore appropriate to a democratic sexuality education, can be clarified by examining differing ideological positions toward homosexuality in terms of their acceptability as a basis for education or social policy in a society governed by the overlapping consensus of a liberal democracy.

In *Virtually Normal: An Argument About Homosexuality*, Andrew Sullivan (1995) sketches four different positions on homosexuality—the prohibitionist, the conservative, the liberationist, the liberal—each with a "distinct solution to the problem of gay-straight relations" (p. 20). As we might infer from these labels, the prohibitionist and conservative positions are encompassed by Restrictive sexual ideology and the liberationist and liberal positions reflect Permissive sexual ideology. Each of these perspectives, perhaps with the exception of the liberationist, is sometimes proposed as an appropriate moral framework for addressing the issue of homosexuality in sexuality education. Sullivan describes and critiques each perspective from a philosophical position that is essentially consistent with the conception of democracy explicated by Rawls (1993).

The first perspective that Sullivan delineates is the prohibitionist argument. Its contours are now familiar to us. It is synonymous with the Jehovanist ideology described by Davis (1983) in that it argues on the basis of divine revelation and/or natural law "that homosexuality is an abberation and that homosexual acts are an abomination" (Sullivan, 1995, p. 20). Thus, homosexuality, in this view, requires legal punishment and social deterrence.

Because this conceptualization of homosexuality has enjoyed a relative hegemony throughout most of the history of Western culture, its moral prescriptions have been codified in law and have permeated our culture, including formal and informal attempts at public education about sexuality. In terms of the law, the hegemony of this perspective towards homosexuality has resulted in the codification of a particular sexual ideology into the legal regulation of sexual behaviour. Ruse (1988), equating the prohibitionist perspective toward homosexuality with the tenets of the Christian tradition, summarizes this marriage of a specific moral world view with the legal regulation of society.

> I doubt that anyone has wanted (or today would want) to equate moral law exactly with legal law. Nevertheless, in the past many have clearly seen a close connection between sins (violations of moral laws) and crimes (violations of state laws). People have felt that inasmuch as possible the state law ought to uphold the moral law, legislating against sin, and in turn being supported by the moral law. Furthermore, in the west moral law has been seen in turn to be part and parcel of the Christian tradition. (p. 241)

In sum, Restrictive sexual ideology, at least with respect to homosexuality, has been, and to a considerable extent continues to be, the law of the land.

If we transpose this dynamic to sexuality education we can suppose that the substance of the moral law (homosexual acts are an abomination) is merged with the content of sexuality education with the result that students are unequivocally told that homosexual acts are immoral.

For some fairly clear reasons, this approach, in both its legal and educational implications, is at odds with Rawls' (1993) conceptualization of democracy and with a democratic philosophy of sexuality education. In Rawlsian terms, the prohibitionist perspective toward homosexuality, as a moral belief, constitutes part of a comprehensive doctrine. To the extent that the prohibitionist view is imposed on the members of society, either in terms of law or the process of education, it constitutes what Rawls (1993) calls an unreasonable doctrine. It is in violation of the overlapping consensus upon which democratic society is based.

The second perspective that Sullivan (1995) describes that falls under the rubric of Restrictive sexual ideology is the conservative approach to homosexuality. Sullivan's (1995) conservative category mirrors, in many ways, Seidman's (1992) description of Romanticist sexual ideology which stresses the ideal of mature heterosexual unions. According to Sullivan (1995), conservatives disapprove of homosexuality

> because homosexual sex cannot partake of the uniquely heterosexual union of procreation and emotional commitment that loving straight marital sex can partake in; and because its simulation of such an act is simply a delusion on the part of those involved. (p. 99)

In short, in this view, homosexuality is psychologically unhealthy and constitutes an affront to mature heterosexuality. According to Sullivan (1995), although conservatives share a basic respect for democratic principles, they advocate the guiding of public life to reflect their view of healthy sexuality.

> Conservatives combine a private tolerance of homosexuals with public disapproval of homosexuality. While they do not want to see legal persecution of homosexuals, they see no problem with discouragement and disparagement of homosexual behavior in the abstract or, more commonly, a carefully sustained hush on the matter altogether. (p. 97)[2]

Social policy, then, is geared toward discouraging "all public messages that undermine the exclusively marital, heterosexual, and loving deployment of sexual desire" (Ibid., p. 101).

Although the conservatives, unlike the prohibitionists, do not favour legal measures to prevent homosexual acts from occurring, conservative social policy still constitutes an unreasonable doctrine. We can assume that a conservative sexuality education would actively seek to promote "the exclusively marital, heterosexual, and loving deployment of sexual desire." It is difficult to imagine that sexuality education of this sort could possibly avoid being justifiably labelled as indoctrination. As Rawls (1993) emphasizes, categorizing a doctrine as unreasonable does not imply that the doctrine's stance on a particular moral issue is invalid, but rather it is the attempt to impose that moral stance that may render the doctrine unreasonable. Clearly, on these grounds, the conservative social policy towards homosexuality, and, by extension, its approach to addressing homosexuality in sexuality education, constitutes an unreasonable doctrine.

The third approach to homosexuality described by Sullivan (1995) is the liberationist. The point of departure for the liberationist approach is a strain of the social constructionist analysis of sexuality that was outlined in detail in Chapter Four. In its more extreme forms it suggests that our prevailing concepts of gender and sexual orientation are nothing but socially created categories; "a particular way of being as defined by a particular culture" (Sullivan, 1995, p. 58).

> For the liberationists, homosexuality as a defining condition does not properly exist because it is a construct of human thought, not an inherent or natural state of being. It is a "construction," generated in human consciousness by the powerful to control and define the powerless. It reflects not the true state of human affairs, but a crude and arbitrary ordering imposed upon them. As with many prohibitionists, there are no homosexuals, merely same-sex acts; only unlike the prohibitionists, even these acts are dependant on their social context for their meaning. (Ibid., p. 57)

As I suggested in Chapter Four, the social constructionist analysis can lead us to an acknowledgement, and perhaps affirmation, of a plurality of sexual meanings. However, the liberationists described by Sullivan (1995) attach to the social constructionist analysis a politics that seeks to promote a version of Permissive sexual ideology. In other words, rather than affirm diversity by placing existing categories of gender and sexual orientation on an equal footing, the liberationist prescribes that these categories must be obliterated. The elimination of these categories reflects Permissive sexual ideology because those groups who suffer oppression under prevailing categorizations, particularly women and homosexuals, will presumably enjoy greater sexual freedom once gender and sexual orientation no longer exist as meaningful categories. When this view is translated into a prescription, insisting that public institutions must preside over the destruction of prevailing constructions of gender and sexual orientation, it becomes an unreasonable doctrine. It is in fact a proposal to impose a particular conception of the human condition on people, many of whom may not think it possible or even desirable, including, it should be noted, many women and homosexuals.

The fourth perspective toward homosexuality outlined by Sullivan (1995) is the modern liberal interpretation. This perspective is best described as modern because it strays from, and in many ways contradicts, the principles of traditional liberalism. This distinction is important and worth articulating in some detail because it allows us to see that the modern liberal approach to homosexuality violates the principles of liberal democracy articulated by Rawls (1993). It is also reflects how a modern liberal sexuality education may skew instruction in favour of Permissive sexual ideology.

According to Sullivan (1995),

> there is a line over which a liberal citizen will not cross; he or she refuses to see the state as a way to inculcate virtue or to promote one way of living over another; the state has no role in promoting understanding or compassion or tolerance, as opposed to toleration, or indeed to celebrate one set of "values" over another; and where the state and the individual conflict, the liberal will almost always side with the individual. (p. 139)

For example, in order to combat discrimination against racial minorities, traditional liberals favoured political remedies such as ensuring voting rights, equal protection of the law, and equal access to education and public services.

> But insofar as they were subject to more elusive social pressures—social prejudice, snobbery, racial bigotry, ridicule, nonviolent sexual harassment—liberals were content to illuminate the injustice, persuade others not to practice it, and to make their case relentlessly in the forums of liberal society: in literature, journalism, theatre, and the visual arts, in the mass media, and elsewhere. Injustice in the state, liberals believed, should be abolished; injustice in civil society should be admonished. (Sullivan, 1995, p. 146)

In its contemporary incarnation, however, Sullivan (1995) detects that liberalism has strayed from these principles. This deviation was, according to Sullivan (1995), well intentioned. It was a consequence of the fact that abolishing injustice in the state and merely admonishing it in civil life was largely ineffective. Despite the hopes of a liberal society, inequality and injustice stubbornly persist as features of Western culture. In response to this reality, according to Sullivan (1995), liberalism began to betray itself by breaching the principle of public neutrality. Toward the end of the 20th century, "liberalism extended itself into other, more far reaching areas of morals and social meaning" (p. 141). To promote liberty and equality in these private spheres required that limitations were to be put on what once were liberalism's sacred principles.

According to Sullivan (1995), antidiscrimination statutes informed by this contemporary incarnation of liberalism reveal a contradiction. That is, in order to create an environment of equality for minority groups, liberals were forced to curtail the majority's right to liberty. In other words, these statutes

> are designed not simply to protect the rights of a minority, but to educate a backward majority in the errors of its ways. It is perhaps no wonder that in the arena of public debate, liberals have found themselves increasingly undermined by their own tradition. (Sullivan, 1995, p. 137)

"In its original, ideal formulation, liberalism could always assert that it was completely neutral in its dealings between citizens....But now the state was becoming intimately involved in the details of *private* life" (Ibid., p. 143).

According to Sullivan (1995), in relation to its goal of promoting equality for homosexuals, contemporary liberalism has fallen victim to this paradox. Sullivan (1995), argues that "the modern liberal is so concerned to overcome the visceral hostility toward homosexuals in the society that he wishes to reduce all of these emotions to a binary bigoted-tolerant axis, and legislate in favor of the tolerant" (p. 151). Further, laws designed to accomplish this goal are "forced into being a mixture of moral education, psychotherapy, and absolution. Liberalism was invented specifically to oppose this use of the law" (Ibid.).

To the extent that Sullivan's critique of modern liberalism is correct, that approach contradicts Rawls' (1993) conception of political liberalism.

The contemporary liberal approach to homosexuality, as described by Sullivan, constitutes an unreasonable doctrine in that it attempts to legislate away the beliefs of those who oppose homosexuality. While this approach is clearly noble in its aspiration to achieve a general standing of equality for homosexuals in society, the means by which this goal is to be achieved runs afoul of the principles of political Liberalism.

This concern, articulated by Sullivan, about the intrusiveness of contemporary liberalism has implications for how sexuality education addresses the issue of homosexuality. Many sexuality educators are keenly aware of the discrimination, hatred, and violence faced by homosexuals by virtue of their sexual orientation. Some may be tempted to respond to this state of affairs by condemning as incorrect the expression of any view opposed to homosexuality. In other words, the response may be to teach from a position of exclusive partiality, insisting, for example, that homosexuality must be accepted by students as morally valid. When we take this route, a curious paradox becomes evident. The belief that homosexual behaviour is immoral is part of a comprehensive doctrine that has considerable currency in our culture. If we demand its suppression, an appeal to democratic principles in advocating the equal expression of perspectives that affirm homosexuality collapses in contradiction. How can we argue for the expression of gay and lesbian positive perspectives in public schools, particularly those that exist in communities that are largely hostile to these views, when we simultaneously argue that those who believe that homosexuality is wrong have no right to express their own conceptions of the good moral life? Democratic principles will offer us little help if moral indoctrination is our apparatus for achieving an inclusive curriculum. We must be very clear in arguing for sexuality education that promotes gay and lesbian rights that we have no desire for moral engineering other than to promote the democratic right to moral autonomy. The aim of a democratic sexuality education is not to establish which values are objectively superior in regard to homosexuality, but rather to have students consider different moral positions in the context of democratic society. However, it must be made crystal clear that while the public school should not be used as a vehicle to impose or reject the moral affirmation of homosexual behaviour, it must, if it is to contribute to a democratic society, promote and respect the rights of homosexuals.

It might be argued that to discuss and debate the moral validity of same-sex sexuality is itself a form of discrimination since the moral validity of heterosexuality is rarely, if ever, seriously contested. Although this position may have some merit in a philosophical sense, the moral validity of homosexuality needs to be addressed in a democratic sexuality education because, whether one likes it or not, it is an issue that divides our society. Refusing to allow the issue to be brought up for discussion on the grounds that it constitutes discrimination to do so will not make the issue go away. It will only leave prevailing moral norms, some of which are clearly discriminatory, unexamined.

It is true that within a democratic culture, each of us is fully entitled to believe whatever we may wish with respect to the morality of homosexual behaviour. It is equally true, however, that in a democratic society, each of us is duty bound by the overlapping consensus of basic values to fully respect the freedom of all individuals in our society to pursue their own conception of the good life provided they do not infringe on the rights of others. The implications of this for the way in which a democratic society addresses the rights of homosexuals should easily be deduced. The fact that considerable uncertainty and debate continues to exist about gay and lesbian rights is a compelling example of how sexual ideology has supplanted democratic principles as a guiding force in much of the public discourse on this issue. Here we are provided with what are perhaps the most vivid examples of where lower order sexual ideology is the basis for public policy both in the society at large and subsequently in sexuality education in the schools. While much of the contemporary debate around homosexuality is couched in legal terms, it is important to recognize that, at its essence, it is not simply the legal status of homosexuals that is at question but what conceptions of the good life will be affirmed by the state. A philosophy of sexuality education, like other forms of public policy, ought to be guided by the principles of the overlapping consensus of a liberal democracy in which multiple conceptions of the good life are affirmed.

Whether or not one morally approves or disapproves of homosexual behaviour is immaterial to the principle inherent within a democratic society that all people, irrespective of their sexual orientation or other such characteristic, have the inalienable right to live a life free of discrimination. This points us to the straightforward principle that "discrimination against homosexuals be ended and that every right and responsibility that heterosexuals enjoy as public citizens be extended to those who grow up and find themselves emotionally different" (Sullivan, 1995, p. 171). Extending these rights to gays and lesbians in no way subverts the rights of those who find

homosexuality morally problematic, it only allows for those who are homosexual to enjoy the basic rights which the overlapping consensus of a
democratic culture must grant to all people.

It is well documented that homosexuals are often the victims of various
forms of legal discrimination because of their sexual orientation. In 1986,
in *Bowers v. Hardwick*, the United States supreme court ruled that the states
had the right to make homosexual sex between consenting adults a crime.
As a result, 32 states have laws forbidding homosexual sodomy (Swan, 1997).
Thus, for all intents and purposes, homosexual sex, even if it is between
consenting adults in the privacy of their own home, is illegal. From the
perspective of a liberal democracy this can be seen as nothing less than the
unwarranted use of the law to impose a sexual ideology. In 11 states, courts
have ruled that gays and lesbians are unfit to have custody of their children.
Only one state, Hawaii, recognizes same-sex marriages (Swan, 1997). In
Canada, the legal status of homosexuals is comparatively better. In 1996,
discrimination on the basis of sexual orientation was prohibited by the
Canadian Human Rights Act and in 1969 homosexual sex between consenting adults was decriminalized. Still, marriages between homosexuals are not
legally recognized in Canada and recent initiatives to extend spousal benefits to same sex couples have been defeated by provincial legislatures (Barrett
et al., 1997). In the province of Alberta, homosexuals have recently been
barred from being foster parents (Mitchell & Laghi, 1997).

As with many other controversial issues, public school sexuality education has tended toward exclusion rather than inclusion with respect to the
way it addresses sexual orientation. However, this tendency is more
pernicious than the exclusive neutrality that is characteristic of so much
contemporary sexuality education. In many cases, the absence of homosexuality in the sexuality education curriculum represents a wilful attempt
to marginalize or ignore any conceptualization of human sexuality that does
not fit the heterosexual norm. In some places in the United States,
discussion of the topic is banned from the formal curriculum. For example,
in South Carolina, legislators have banned discussion of homosexuality in
the formal curriculum except within the context of a class discussion about
AIDS (Sears, 1992, p. 139). Concerted and deliberate attempts to remove
sexual orientation issues from the school curriculum have recently occured
in New York City, Des Moines, Iowa, and the state of California (for a review
of these controversies see Phariss, 1997). Barrett et al. (1997) note that

"Canadian schools have been slow to introduce adequate discussion of gay and lesbian sexuality in school curricula, and those who attempt to do so often encounter strong opposition from organized groups from the religious right" (p. 276). Not only do these attempts to censor sexuality education curricula deny students the opportunity for critical deliberation, such censorship blatantly discriminates against gay and lesbian students for the simple reason that their educational needs are effectively dismissed as nonexistent or irrelevant. Sexuality educators need to make every effort to ensure that the educational needs of gay and lesbian youth are accorded equal respect and appropriate attention. Secondly, educators must recognize that gay and lesbian adolescents face extraordinary challenges not faced by heterosexual teenagers. They are frequently the targets of harassment and violence by their peers. They often have difficulty dealing with disapproving parents. They face the often disconcerting, if not outright terrifying, prospect of revealing their identity to others. In short, as Martin (1988) states "The truth is that gay and lesbian youth are not like other adolescents. Their difference stems from their status as members of one of the most hated and despised minority groups in the country" (p. 59). While educators cannot eliminate hostile beliefs toward homosexuals, it is their duty, as part of the responsibility of providing a democratic sexuality education, to do their best to ensure that gay and lesbian adolescents are accorded an equal dignity and respect both inside and outside the classroom.

It is estimated that more than 90% of gay men and lesbians are the targets of verbal abuse or threats and more than one third are the victims of violence related to their sexual orientation (Fassinger, 1991). These statistics clearly reflect a widespread assault on the basic democratic rights of homosexuals. Two tendencies are at work in contributing to this violation of homosexual rights in contemporary society. In both cases, sexuality education has an important role to play in promoting the basic rights of homosexuals.

The first tendency is for people to translate their moral disapproval of homosexuality into a rationale and justification for infringing on the rights of homosexuals. Clearly, within the bounds of the overlapping consensus of a democratic society's basic values, such a linkage is untenable. For a democratic sexuality education, the message to students is unambigious. While we are free in a democratic society to morally approve or disapprove of particular sexual acts, discrimination, even against those whose behaviour we may personally find morally wanting, is contrary to the principles of democracy. To disapprove morally of homosexuality is to believe that sexual acts between members of the same sex are wrong in the ethical sense. Discrimination is the negative differential treatment of individuals or groups based on criteria that include race, class, disability, religion, gender, and sexual orientation. Negative differential treatment based on such criteria inevitably prevents people with these characteristics from freely pursuing the good life as they conceive it. The concept of democracy supports the right to freedom of belief which includes the right to disapprove morally of another person's lifestyle but at the same time unequivocally distinguishes this right from, and rejects, attempts to impose a particular conception of the good life on others. This distinction is important because while a genuinely democratic society encourages respect for diversity and formally prohibits discrimination, it does not dictate moral values (McKay & Barrett, 1995). Understanding and acting upon this distinction is an essential component of a functioning democracy. Given the prevalence of discrimination based on sexual orientation in our society, sexuality education can, by addressing this issue, promote the democratic right to equality for gays and lesbians. One of the primary virtues of a democratic sexuality education is that because it makes democratic principles the foundation and substance of curriculum content it is structured so that the distinction between the lower order approval or disapproval of particular sexual acts and the higher order obligation to respect the freedom of others to follow their own conception of the good life is continually emphasized and examined.

A second major contributor to the violation of gay and lesbian rights, and therefore an important issue for sexuality education to address, is homophobia. Homophobia is, by definition, not a moral or political term. The term homophobia is properly used to describe a psychological state. As Celia Kitzinger (1996) puts it, "the word *homophobia* derives from (and is used within) the academic discipline of psychology: *phobia* comes from the Greek for 'fear', as in claustrophobia or agoraphobia, meaning an irrational fear or dread" (p. 8). There can be no doubt that this irrational fear or dread is a leading contributor to the violence and palpable ostracism that so many homosexuals face. The propensity on the part of individuals and institutions to discriminate against homosexuals can, therefore, be at least partially reduced once the irrational fear of gays and lesbians is, itself, alleviated.

Education has a key role in reducing homophobia because much of this irrational fear is based on myth and ignorance. For example, some homophobes seem to believe that gays and lesbians are interested in "recruiting" heterosexuals into the homosexual fold or that homosexuality is "contagious" or that gay men are more likely than heterosexual men to be child molestors. Since none of these beliefs are accurate, sexuality education, by providing basic information about the topic, can help to dispel these myths. However, for many if not most homophobes, the irrational fear of homosexuals is emotionally rather than cognitively based. This is most readily seen in the homophobic tendancies of high school age males who seem to have a particularly pronounced disdain toward homosexuality. A study using a nationally representative sample of 15- to 19-year-old males in the United States found that 89% of the sample indicated that they thought that men having sex with men was "disgusting" and 59% felt they would be unable to be friends with a gay person (Marsiglio, 1993). It is perhaps not surprising that such feelings might arise at a time when most adolescent males are highly focussed on their own sense of masculinity, something they are anxious to assert to themselves and to others. Showing disdain for homosexuals functions as a way for the teenage boy to convince both himself and others that he is conventionally masculine. In the Marsiglio (1993) study it was found that young men with more traditional male gender role attitudes were significantly more likely to have negative attitudes toward homosexuality. In sum, many homophobic men may be attempting to reaffirm their male identity by verbally or physically attacking homosexuals. Beyond dispelling myths and emphasizing the rights and responsibilities of democratic living, sexuality education, if it is to contribute to the reduction of homophobia in our society, must also address the dimensions of homophobia which are psychologically rooted. Part of this process involves having students critically examine male gender roles and the meaning of masculinity.

Based on the principles of a democratic sexuality education, teaching about the issue of sexual orientation should be guided by the following considerations. First, despite arguments about the actual numbers of gays, lesbians, and bisexuals in the general population, the fact remains that the average classroom will be characterized by at least some degree of diversity with respect to sexual orientation. Figures on the prevalence of homosexuality reported in the scientific literature or in the media depend on whether it is behaviour, desire, or identity that is being reported. In the most comprehensive probability-based survey of sexual behaviour ever done in the United States, 9% of women and 10% of men over the age of 18 reported some degree of homosexual behaviour, desire, or identity (Lauman et al., 1994). In general, research on the prevalence of homosexuality suggests that between 5% to 10% of the population is not heterosexual (for a review of this research see Michaels, 1997). Even if we use a very conservative estimate that 5% of the population is either gay, lesbian or bisexual, this means that a classroom with 20 or more students is likely to have at least one student who is not heterosexual. If sexuality education is to try to meet the educational needs of all of its students, it cannot avoid teaching about diverse sexualities. Michael Reiss (1997), in discussing the issue of addressing sexual orientation in schools in the United Kingdom, draws the analogy that

> while homosexuals are undeniably a minority, they are a sizable one—comparable, in the United Kingdom, to the number of Muslims or Roman Catholics. As such they deserve the attention and curriculum space when teaching sex education that should be accorded to religious minorities when teaching religious education. (p. 344)

An additional consideration is that gay, lesbian, and bisexual youth grow up in a culture that is normatively heterosexual and as a result the opportunities for these young people to learn about their own sexuality is greatly reduced. As a result, their need for sexuality education may be even more significant, particularly in communities where homosexuality is largely invisible.

Secondly, a democratic sexuality education helps students to clarify their own values with respect to sexual orientation. Student opinions will be dependent on many factors including the values that they have already brought with them to the classroom. The family, peers, religious authorities, the media and other sources of knowledge and value perspectives will have inevitably informed students' knowledge and opinions about homosexuality. A democratic sexuality education will encourage students to clarify their own value positions toward sexual orientation and compare them to the best arguments put forth by various ideological perspectives. This process of critical deliberation can contribute meaningfully to the knowledgable and critical appropriation of value perspectives. For example, young people need to have knowledge that according to some religious traditions homosexuality is seen as a sin, and just as significantly, they need to learn that the overwhelming consensus of contemporary psychology is that homosexuality is a healthy sexual orientation. Such an exercise not only facilitates critical deliberation, it promotes understanding between students with different points of view and different sexual orientations.

> For instance, a heterosexual student might gain some idea of what it is like to be homosexual in a society where most people assume you are not, while a homosexual student from an agnostic background might gain some idea of what it might be like to be brought up in a family with strong religious beliefs which include the view that homosexual behaviour is completely unacceptable. (Reiss, 1997, p. 347)

Thirdly, sexuality education that promotes democratic principles addresses the issue of sexual orientation, first and foremost, in terms of the overlapping consensus of democratic values. In this respect, the issue for a democratic sexuality education is not whether homosexual behaviour is right or wrong. Rather, the objective is first to understand differing perspectives and second to think about how such views can co-exist in a democratic culture that not only respects freedom of belief but also promotes democratic values of liberty, justice, and equality. It encourages students to use the criteria of the overlapping consensus of democracy to critically evaluate various perspectives toward homosexuality. Furthermore, if it is to embody democratic values, sexuality education must promote the rights of gays, lesbians, and bisexuals. This involves not only examining the basic values of democracy but also actively working against homophobia.

Promoting Gender Equality Through Sexuality Education

Given that our society categorizes and defines us along lines of gender, there can be little doubt that the social organization of relations between the genders has a monumental impact on each of our lives and on the nature of society itself. Clearly, sexual behaviour is gendered behaviour, including "expectations about how men and women are supposed to behave in sexual situations" (Byers, 1991, p. 16) and this may be particularly the case in adolescent relationships (Mackie, 1987).

As was suggested in Chapters One and Two, there are deep ideological divisions about the sources of male-female differences related to sexuality and what constitutes an appropriate organization of gender relations within society. For example, Restrictive sexual ideology, with the exception of Radical feminism, tends to favour what can best be described as traditional gender roles, whereas Permissive sexual ideology tends to argue for a more progressive and transformative approach to gender relations. However, prevailing ideological divisions related to gender cannot be reduced to a straightforward opposition between the Permissive and Restrictive sexual ideologies. It is evident that within the feminist movement itself, there are also deep divisions related to the desired transformation of gender relations within society (e.g., McCormick, 1994). The link between gender and sexuality, combined with intense ideological divisions over the proper direction of gender relations, raises important issues for the form and content of sexuality education.

First, we need to be clear on the extent to which gender relations are shaped by ideology. A number of social scientists have proposed that many gender attributes related to sexuality are the products of biological and psychological adaptations acquired through the processes of human evolution (e.g., Buss, 1994; Symons, 1979). Be that as it may, there is little question, even among psychobiologists, that the arrangement of gender relations within a given society entails a series of social constructs. These social constructs result from ideologically based assumptions about what it means to be a man or woman, the roles each plays in society, and how men and women ought to relate to each other. That these assumptions are socially constructed is made evident by the fact that they are the subject of considerable variation and elasticity from one historical period to another and from one culture to another. As Connell (1987) aptly puts it,

> Social-scientific theories of gender are a Western invention, as far as I know, and definitely a modern one. Other civilizations have had their own ways of dealing with human sexuality and the relations between the sexes. As Indian eroticism and Chinese family codes illustrate, these can be as sophisticated and elaborate as anything the West has created. But they are different kinds of cultural formation. (p. 23)

In particular, it is the relationship between the genders that is determined by a given society's social structure. In Connell's (1987) words, "Gender relations involve the structuring of social practice around sex and sexuality" (p. 245). I have argued that the structuring of social practice around sexuality, and our beliefs about it, are dependant on our ideological predispositions. In this respect, the issues surrounding the debate on gender equality are issues of ideology. For example, as Connell (1987) notes, when the 19th century feminist Mary Wollstonecraft advocated the rights of women "it was mainly questions of ideology she had in mind: morals, manners, education and religion" (p. 241).

If the interconnection between sexuality and gender relations is a matter of ideology, we might expect that sexuality education in the schools would, at the very least, make students aware of an ideological analysis of gender relations. Sexuality education, at virtually any grade level, that invites students to consider the role of gender in sexual relationships without reference to differing ideological assumptions related to gender relations, is either highly deceptive in its own ideological bias or reflects an extreme exclusive neutrality.

The manner in which most prevailing forms of sexuality education in the schools approach gender relations is suggestive of what Connell (1987) calls "the cognitive purification of the world of gender" (p. 346). In other words, gender relations, when they are discussed at all, are not presented as something subject to social construction and transformation, but rather patterns of gender relations are presented as accepted but unquestioned facts. As Connell (1987) notes, "The interpretation of gender relations as natural facts is extraordinarily widespread" (p. 245). In addition, these "natural facts" of gender relations tend to reflect very traditional assumptions about the gendered aspects of sexual relationships. As I have noted, many feminists identify these traditional assumptions as important factors in the oppression of women.

A number of authors have observed that contemporary sexuality education presents a traditional picture of gender relations that remains largely uncritiqued (Fine, 1988; Lenskyj, 1990; Sapon-Shevin & Goodman, 1992; Szirom, 1988; Whatley, 1988). For example, Fine (1988), in her study of sexuality education in urban American schools, observed that programs often address adolescent female sexuality solely in terms of the threat of aggressive male sexuality. This kind of sexuality education presupposes as "natural facts" the traditional gender scripts of male sexual aggressiveness and female sexual passivity. The *Sex Respect* and *Teen-Aid* curriculums have been criticized on the grounds that they perpetuate a stereotypical and male-biased pattern of gender relations (Whatley & Trudell, 1993). In sum, sexuality education often reinforces traditional patterns of gender relations by implicitly, if not explicitly, encouraging young women and men to view themselves as living embodiments of the "natural facts" of gender relations.

It is unlikely that sexuality education based on the "natural facts" of gender relations can contribute to the understanding of the social construction of gender relations or to the critical deliberation between differing ideological perspectives toward gender and sexuality. If these are necessary ingredients for the promotion of gender equality in sexuality education, prevailing forms of sexuality education are likely to contribute little to this endeavour.

Szirom (1988) argues that

> Neither the theories advanced by the proponents of sex education, nor the most used teaching materials on which these courses are based, have addressed the fundamental issues of sex differences in socialization and the repression of women's sexuality; they are still therefore, inherently sexist in orientation. (p. xxi)

Assuming that a purposeful quest for gender equality in sexuality and other realms is a widely shared and justifiable goal in a democratic society, it is necessary to conceptualize the manner in which a democratic sexuality education addresses this issue. When we speak of promoting gender equality in sexuality education we are, by definition, talking about bringing a feminist perspective to the classroom. It is the feminist movement that promotes women's interests with the aim of achieving equality with men. However, this begs the question, how can a feminist approach to sexuality education avoid the imposition of ideological assumptions related to gender and gender relations? This question is particularly vexing since the feminist movement itself encompasses a wide range of ideological perspectives.

I will focus here on the issue of ideological diversity within the feminist movement, and not on an opposition between feminist and antifeminist perspectives, because I am presupposing that a feminist approach to sexuality education is legitimate in-so-far as feminism is, broadly speaking, devoted to promoting the interests of women in a world that has been, and is, largely ruled by men. It is, however, important to specify how a feminist sexuality education can remain consistent with the principles of a democratic sexuality education.

The feminist movement as a whole encompasses a variety of ideologies. For example, when we think of Radical feminism, Liberal feminism, or Socialist feminism, we are thinking of specific feminist ideologies, each with their own world views and distinctive analyses of gender relations. However, it may also be said that all feminist ideologies are united in their shared belief in the need to work for and achieve gender equality. It would be a mistake, then, to associate feminism with a specific ideology. Feminist philosopher Janet Radcliffe Richards (1980) proposes a conceptualization of gender along these lines. She suggests that the essence of feminism is the claim that "women suffer from systematic social injustice because of their sex" (pp. 13-14) but that "The conflation of the idea of feminism as a particular ideology with that of feminism as a concern with women's problems" (p. 15) is problematic because it runs the risk of subsuming feminism generally under the rubric of a particular feminist ideology, casting aside other feminist perspectives.

> If feminists themselves think of feminism as the movement which defends women's interests and also as being ideologically committed in a particular direction, the effect will be to fossilize current feminist views...however committed any feminist may be to her ideology she must allow that there is a difference between maintaining the ideology and accepting more generally that women are unjustly treated. (p. 16)

In effect, according to Richards, the broader definition of feminism, distinct from particular feminist ideologies, makes it more plausible for feminism generally to accommodate and be inclusive of a variety of specific feminist ideologies. This is, a useful distinction to make because it provides a way of conceptualizing feminism so that our approach to incorporating issues of gender equality into sexuality education is compatible with a democratic philosophy of education.

With respect to specific feminist ideologies, this implies that no one feminist perspective should be superimposed on the promotion of gender equality in sexuality education. To do so promotes neither critical awareness nor genuine freedom from oppression. From the standpoint of a democratic philosophy of education, replacing the "natural facts" of gender with a specific feminist ideology merely entails the substitution of one set of "facts" for another. If genuine freedom requires the ability to recognize and choose among alternatives, sexuality education cannot be said to promote gender equality in a democratic fashion if it imposes a particular feminist ideology. With respect to feminism generally, Richards (1980) states this approach as follows:

> The true liberator can always be recognized by her wanting to *increase* the options open to the people who are to be liberated, and there is never any justification for taking a choice away from a group you want to liberate unless it is demonstrable beyond all reasonable doubt that removing it will bring other, more important, options into existence. To give women freedom we must give them more choice, and then if

they really do not want the things they are choosing now, like homes and families, those things will just die out without our having to push them. (p. 100)

From a democratic point of view, promoting gender equality through sexuality education involves not imposing a particular ideological perspective of what constitutes gender equality in the sexual realm or how it can be individually or collectively achieved. Rather, promoting gender equality in a democratic sexuality education involves expanding students' critical awareness of the wide range of ideological perspectives on the meaning of gender equality and the best means to reach it for both individuals and society. Fostering critical deliberation in this area represents a rejection of gender relations as "natural facts," A "natural facts" approach or conceptualization of gender relations inhibits freedom of belief because it cannot offer alternatives to itself. It is limited to offering only its own presuppositional lens for thinking about gender relations.

Both the Restrictive and Permissive sexual ideologies offer a wide range of ideological perspectives on gender relations including very different perceptions of the nature of gender, appropriate gender roles, and the meaning of gender equality. This is fertile ground for young people, both men and women, to deliberate critically between competing ideological perspectives toward one of the most important social issues of our time. What do democratic values imply about the current, past, and future shape of gender relations? Unless educators foster critical deliberation on these issues, they not only discourage freedom of belief, they neglect their obligation to develop in young people the capacity to participate, as citizens of a democracy, in a fundamental issue of social justice. As with other issues, social justice related to gender relations is not something that occurs outside the lived experiences and practices of individuals. As Connell (1987) suggests, it "is about change produced by human practice, about people being inside the process" (p. 144). A democratic sexuality education facilitates the ability of young people to become part of the process of achieving gender equality.

Addressing the Issue of Pregnancy/STD Prevention

Of all the controversial issues surrounding sexuality education, the question of how best to help adolescents avoid unwanted pregnancy and infection with STDs, including HIV/AIDS, is one of the most widely debated. Indeed, within the contemporary public and professional discourse on sexuality education, the ability to influence teenage behaviour effectively for the purposes of pregnancy/STD prevention is the gold standard by which sexuality education programs are ultimately judged.

Like other aspects of health education, sexuality education has become increasingly driven by a behaviour modification agenda. Morris (1994, pp. 15-23) argues that many sexuality education programs, in response to the growing awareness of problems of teenage pregnancy, STDs, and especially AIDS, have been reduced to an exercise in crisis-resolution. According to Welle, Russel, and Kittleson (1995), perspectives favouring a "behavior change philosophy in all types of health education settings have inundated professional journals for the past fifteen years" (p. 327). They define a behaviour change philosophy as one that "emphasizes behavioral modifica-tion....Program objectives are quantifiable and measurable" (Welle, Russel, & Kittleson, 1995, p. 327). In regard to pregnancy prevention, Frost and Darroch Forrest (1995) note that

> preventing unintended births to adolescents is politically and socially appealing to everyone. But each time the issue arises, people voice the same questions: "Which interventions work?" "Which programs are the most effective in preventing unintended teenage pregnancies?" "How effective is each program?" "Given different levels of effective-ness and different costs, which programs will give the biggest bang for the buck?" (p. 188)

In this respect, sexuality education has become a means to an end.

Rarely do we hear in the public and professional discourse on adolescent pregnancy/STD prevention questions about whether such programs respect the principles of democratic education: Do these programs impartially encourage students to deliberate critically between the various avenues to pregnancy/STD prevention and their complementary, often value laden, ideological underpinnings? Do these programs genuinely foster the critical appropriation of the often ideologically based decision to be abstinent or to practise safer sex? From even a cursory glance at public school sexuality education in North America it is abundantly clear that these considerations are very often cast aside, sacrificed at the altar of behaviour modification strategies promoting, first and foremost, the Restrictive ideological message that abstinence is best.[3]

In many respects, this approach to sexuality education is under-standable. Unwanted pregnancies and STDs present a major threat to the health and well-being of all people, including teenagers. And, as many social critics are at pains to point out, these problems inflict considerable social and economic costs on society. It is certainly a legitimate objective for sexuality education to attempt to provide young people with the means to prevent themselves from suffering the consequences of unwanted pregnancy and STD infection. Despite the propensity for exclusively partial or exclusively neutral sexuality education in our schools, young people have a right to a meaningful education in this area.

However, from the perspective of a democratic sexuality education, when a behaviour modification approach is subject to direction from sexual ideology, disturbing questions arise. For example, it now seems clear that if educational programs are to have any positive impact on sexual behaviour, they must provide opportunities to acquire the relevant information, motivation, and behavioural skills to avoid sexual health related problems (e.g., see Fisher & Fisher, 1992). For obvious reasons, a presentation of this information, motivation, behavioural skills package, based solely on either Restrictive or Permissive sexual ideology is exclusively partial and therefore undemocratic. Such a presentation is an attempt to influence behaviour, not on the basis of legal rules of conduct, but on the basis of a sexual ideology. Furthermore, as I will explain, by attempting to impose the behavioural codes of a particular sexual ideology, such programs may be counter-productive to the goal of pregnancy/STD prevention.

There can be no doubt that a variety of biological and psychosocial factors influence adolescent sexual behaviour. In particular, the emotionally laden dimensions of sexual activity may play havoc with rational deliberation about appropriate sexual conduct. As Katherine Kelley (1983) notes in her discussion of adolescent sexuality,

> When attempting to make a personal decision about whether to engage in a sexual activity or to use a specific contraceptive, they usually operate spontaneously and emotionally rather than coldly and calculatingly....Even when questions of morality enter the picture, the quick, first reaction based on feelings about the matter can outweigh the unemotional facts of the situation....To the extent that questions of morality concern very important matters for adolescents like whether to engage in a first sexual experience, or to initiate sex with a new partner, or to take steps to avoid an unwanted pregnancy, more emotional, less reasoned, and more self-interested thinking would probably prevail. (p. 134)

It is reasonable to speculate that those young people who have critically appropriated their sexual values, particularly in regard to adolescent sexual behaviour, will be better equipped, both psychologically and philosophically, to employ the appropriate information and skills to protect their sexual health successfully. If critical appropriation leads to a greater likelihood of a meaningful commitment to a particular set of values then it follows that people with such value commitments are likely to incorporate those values into their decision-making. In a culture where people, particularly adolescents, are constantly subjected to a melange of often contradictory messages about sexuality, it should not be surprising that the ready-made behavioural scripts provided by sexuality educators are not easily incorporated into their lives. Without a critically appropriated commitment to the values underlying one or another of the pregnancy/STD prevention behavioural scripts, the failure to practise these scripts becomes more plausible. Successfully negotiating the emotion laden, often conflicted world of interpersonal relationships requires at least some sense of self-efficacy as well as some degree of confidence that what one is doing is congruent with one's own critically appropriated values. Perhaps Fisher (1990, p. 3) is at least partially addressing this point when he suggests that in order for adolescents to learn and practise ways to prevent pregnancy and STDs effectively they must, as a first step in the educational process, come to accept their own sexuality.

Jeffrey Kelly (1995) points out that

> Sexual desire is surely one of the most complicated and least scientifically studied human motives; people often do not understand their own motives concerning sexual behavior and frequently have ambivalent feelings concerning whether or not to have sex at a given time with a given individual. These ambivalent feelings may stem not only from motivations related to sex but also from romantic, emotional, and other feelings concerning the other person. Apart from issues of how to behave assertively in refusing unwanted sexual coercions—a skill that can be taught and practiced...—is the often more difficult issue of helping individuals identify and evaluate their values concerning when they want to become sexually intimate with some other person. (p. 113)

In other words, it may be crucial for individuals to identify and evaluate their values in relation to these issues before they can make a genuine and realistic commitment to engage in behavioural scripts that will help them to avoid STDs and unwanted pregnancies.

From the perspective of a democratic philosophy of sexuality education, the abstinence-only approach provides a particularly clear illustration of the problems associated with a narrowly partial approach to pregnancy/STD prevention. On one hand, such an approach attempts to indoctrinate students into accepting the behavioural codes of Restrictive sexual ideology. On the other hand, such programs may not provide the relevant information, motivation, and behavioural skills for students who do not share that ideology or cannot be convinced of its virtue.[4] This tendency is particularly alarming given the fact that a majority of people become sexually active before the age of 20 (see King et al., 1988; Centers for Disease Control, 1995).

The abstinence-only approach to sexuality education shuts down the opportunity for critical deliberation. It seeks to impose a behavioural script for adolescent behaviour that is consistent with Restrictive sexual ideology. Because these programs obstruct the process of critical deliberation and subsequently the critical appropriation of behavioural scripts for pregnancy/STD prevention, including those focussed on abstinence, it is reasonable to speculate that this tendency may play some role in the apparent failure of abstinence-only programs to have any meaningful impact on adolescent sexual behaviour. As we have seen, values can only be critically appropriated when they are freely chosen from the best arguments of competing points of view, something the abstinence-only approach fails to do. Existing peer-reviewed published data suggest that rigorously evaluated abstinence-only sexuality education programs have been ineffective in prodding students to delay first intercourse (Christopher & Roosa, 1990; Jorgensen, Potts, & Camp, 1993; Roosa & Christopher, 1990). This, despite the fact that immediately after exposure to programs such as *Sex Respect* and *Teen-Aid*, some students are willing to endorse, on a questionnaire, abstinent values (Weed & Jensen, 1993) or agree that they have learned things such as "how to stay away from things that could cause problems for me later" (Olsen et al., 1992, p. 374).

It is worth noting that although very few school-based sexuality education programs of any kind have been shown to modify adolescent sexual behaviour, those that have been successful provided information and skills relevant both for students who are sexually active and for those who are not.[5] In other words, they provided behavioural scripts that were amenable to both Restrictive and Permissive sexual ideology. Whether or not people who have critically appropriated their sexual values, as opposed to simply absorbing them, are more likely to take constructive measures to protect their sexual health needs to be more fully researched.

The debate around pregnancy/STD prevention in the schools brings us back once again to the question of whether or not sexuality education that presents ideological perspectives that may be in opposition to the sexual ideology of many parents will unduly influence young people to reject the moral counsel of their parents. This concern is often stated in the context of a claim that the mere exposure to contraceptive/safer sex information will inevitably destroy the resolve of teenagers from families with Restrictive ideological beliefs, resulting in a quick initiation into premarital intercourse. Accordingly, a young person's ability to choose Restrictive ideology and adhere to its principles will be vanquished by the seductive powers of a few classroom hours devoted to the knowledge and skills needed to practise contraception/safer sex consistently if or when a person becomes sexually active. For behaviour, this assumption appears to be unfounded. Young people who have been exposed to contraceptive/safer sex education are not more likely to become sexually active than those who have not (e.g., see Dawson, 1986; Furstenberg, Moore, & Peterson, 1985; Grunseit & Kippax, 1993; Ku, Sonnenstein, & Pleck, 1992; Marsiglio and Mott, 1986; Wellings et al., 1995; Zelnik & Kim, 1982). The architects of one the few behaviourally effective school-based pregnancy prevention programs write in their evaluation report that

> some parents and educators have wondered whether giving young people information about contraceptives along with support for postponing sexual involvement is too confusing a message. Our data suggest that the two messages are not incompatible. Young people who received instruction from family planning counsellors about human sexuality, including family planning, and advise (sic) from student leaders about postponing sexual involvement used information from each component of the program. Students involved in the program were more likely to both postpone sexual involvement and to use contraceptives when they did have sex than were the no-program group. (Howard & McCabe, 1990, p. 25)[6]

It is also well documented that condom distribution programs for adolescents do not increase rates of sexual activity but do significantly increase condom use among those adolescents who are sexually active (Guttmacher et al., 1997; Sellors, McGraw, & McKinlay, 1994).

The literature and public discourse on sexuality education in the schools is preoccupied with the question: Do our STD and pregnancy prevention programs work? Perhaps we need to reinvent the discussion and begin by asking another question: Do our STD and pregnancy prevention programs promote or inhibit the basic freedoms of democracy? It may be the case that the end result of such a discussion will be sexuality education programs that are not only compatible with the basic values of democracy, but are also better able to help people transform their critically appropriated ideological beliefs about sexuality into effective sexual health problem prevention behaviour.

Conclusion

Our ideological presuppositions related to human sexuality inevitably colour our perspectives toward sexual orientation, gender equality, and pregnancy/STD prevention. Thus, it should come as no surprise that these same presuppositions influence what we would like to see taught about these issues in sexuality education in the schools. The issue of sexual orientation provides a good example of how a wide array of differing ideological presuppositions results in an equally wide array of social policy positions. Because these social policy positions are often drawn from what I have called the *lower order* tenets of specific ideologies, as opposed to the *higher order* concerns of a liberal democratic society, approaching the issue of sexual orientation in sexuality education exclusively from one or another of these positions is inconsistent with the principles of a democratic sexuality education.

Discussion of issues such as sexual orientation and gender inevitably give rise to questions of equality. Assuming that democratic societies are concerned with promoting equality, and that education ought to reflect our vision of a just society, we may also assume that educational institutions are similarly interested in promoting equality. Using the example of gender relations, I have argued that unless education raises awareness of different interpretations of the meaning of equality and fosters critical deliberation between these divergent points of view, education inhibits rather than promotes genuine equality.

Because a major goal of sexuality education is to promote the health of those who receive it, unwanted pregnancy and STD prevention is a central focus of most educational programs. In recent years, HIV/AIDS prevention has become a major priority for sexuality education. As I have tried to show, the objective to reduce the incidence of teenage pregnancy and STDs, particularly HIV/AIDS, has often occurred without meaningful consideration of the democratic principle of freedom of belief. Furthermore, I have speculated that the health promotion aspects of sexuality education may become more behaviourally effective if students are helped to appropriate critically their chosen path to sexual health.

My analyses of these three major content areas of sexuality education contain a common thread. There is a fundamental philosophical inconsistency between the overlapping consensus of common values basic to a liberal democratic society and the typical approaches to sexuality education in the schools. A democratic philosophy of sexuality education will help us to reduce significantly or eliminate this inconsistency.

Notes

1.   Over time, much of the terminology related to sexuality, and sexual orientation in particular, has become politicized. I use such terms in a value-neutral way that defines *homosexuality* as a sexual attraction toward another person of the same sex and *homosexual* as a person who is sexually attracted to members of the same sex.

2.   It is worth noting, on this point, that the *Sex Respect* and *Teen-Aid* sexuality education programs, both informed exclusively by Restrictive sexual ideology, are largely silent on the subject of sexual orientation. Homosexuality and homosexual behaviour are only discussed in the context of HIV transmission. Perhaps this is reflective of the conservative strategy of "a carefully sustained hush on the matter" described by Sullivan.

3.   I refer the reader back to the footnote on p. 91 where the association between the "abstinence is best" message and Restrictive sexual ideology is more fully examined.

4.   It may also be argued that while having sexually restrictive attitudes is correlated with more conservative patterns of sexual behaviour, for example having fewer sexual partners, since this correlation does not hold, in many cases, for age of first intercourse, abstinence-only sexuality education may not be fully relevant even to those students who maintain a Restrictive sexual ideology. For example, Laumann et al., (1994) note in their survey of American sexual behaviours and attitudes that many Americans disapprove of teenage sex "even if the respondents themselves reported an early onset of sexual intercourse in their own lives. These views are, apparently, increasingly inconsistent with the actual pattern of behavior" (p. 322). Janus and Janus (1993, p. 252) found in their survey that although there is a negative

correlation between religiosity and the likelihood of having premarital sex, of their respondents who described themselves as "very religious" only 29% reported that they had no sexual experience before marriage. Allgeier (1983) argues that such people may have "ideological barriers" to the use of contraceptives, resulting in an increased likelihood of unintended pregnancy once they become sexually active. Given the apparent frequency of an inconsistency between ideology and behaviour as it relates to premarital sexual activity in particular, from a pregnancy/STD prevention perspective, it can be reasonably argued that abstinence-only sexuality education is not fully relevant even to those students who hold a Restrictive sexual ideology.

5.   For a comprehensive review of this literature see Kirby et al., 1994.

6.   It should be noted that the data I have presented in regard to these questions may be disputed by some people on the grounds that these research studies are based on research paradigms that are biased in support of Permissive sexual ideology (e.g., see the Davis quote on p. 102). Nevertheless, this should not prevent this body of evidence from being introduced into the public policy debate on sexuality education.

Conclusion: Sexuality Education
and Social Justice

A key litmus test for any philosophy of education is whether or not its principles and practices contribute to the social development of society. Ozmon and Craver (1986) suggest that "A philosophy of education becomes significant at the point where educators recognize the need to think clearly about what they are doing and to see what they are doing in the larger context of individual and social development" (p. x). In other words, a philosophy of education has implications that extend beyond the classroom. When a philosophy of education becomes the operating framework from which the socialization of youth into the broader culture takes place, it takes on a significant role in shaping the fabric of the culture itself. Thus, it is logical and legitimate to evaluate the degree to which a given philosophy of education is consistent with the ethos of the culture that it perpetuates and, at times, transforms. This is, ultimately, a question we must pose about any proposed philosophy to guide sexuality education in the schools.

I have tried to make clear that our beliefs and customs related to sexuality are crucial defining characteristics of our culture. I have also suggested that the socialization process of young people in regard to sexuality, through the public education system, must inevitably reflect, to some extent, our attitudes towards sexuality in the larger culture. In other words, how we educate youth about sexuality reflects how we believe people should conduct themselves as members of society. This involves much more than learning how to avoid unwanted pregnancies and STDs or learning how to have satisfying interpersonal relationships. As important as these aspects of sexuality education are, if we are to become functioning members of a democratic society, we must also learn how to co-exist peacefully with those who hold different values about sexuality than our own. It is only when, as educators, we pursue these goals that we can genuinely say that our philosophy of sexuality education reflects a democratic vision of a just society.

As I attempted to show in Chapter Two, in terms of sexuality, Western culture is fractured by deeply seated ideological conflict which I have generalized into the opposition between the Restrictive and Permissive sexual ideologies. Given my assumptions about the basic ethos of a democratic society, as I articulated it in Chapter Four, this clash of ideas is to be expected as the natural outcome of reason under the conditions of freedom in a democratic culture.

However, if education is to reflect and contribute to our vision of the good society, that is our commitment to the democratic ethos, the current state of sexuality education in the schools should give us cause for concern. As I tried to show in Chapter Three, prevailing forms of sexuality education typically do not respect the core democratic principle of freedom of belief and they also typically do not provide an intellectual framework for democratic citizenship in the sense of helping students develop the capacity to participate, in a fashion consistent with the ethos of democracy, in the ongoing debates and conflicts around sexuality that will persist into the future. As Mosher, Kenny, and Garrod (1994) point out, there is a long-standing and widespread agreement that public schools have a duty to foster "the development of youth who understand, value, and enact democracy" (p. 25). Or as John Dewey succinctly says,

> Whether the education process is carried on in a predominately democratic or nondemocratic way becomes, therefore, a question of transcendent importance not only for education itself but for its final effect upon all the interests and activities of a society that is committed to the democratic way of life. (Dewey cited in Mosher, Kenny, & Garrod, 1994, p. 36)

If it is true that "as sex goes, so goes society," providing a sexuality education based on democratic principles is an extremely important endeavour.

In response to the pervasive ideological conflict surrounding sexuality and sexuality education, I have proposed a philosophy of sexuality education based on the overlapping consensus of very limited but common values abstracted from the background culture of a society that affirms moral pluralism. Specifically, I have focussed on the commonly held overlapping consensus in support of the right to freedom of belief, something I have tried to show is often not respected in contemporary forms of sexuality education in the schools. By implication, I have argued that a philosophy of sexuality education based on political liberalism contributes to a just society.

Thus, it is perhaps necessary to discuss why, given the many critiques recently launched against the liberal tradition in politics and philosophy, a democratic theory of education informed by political liberalism is, at this point in history, an approach that contributes to social justice. Will a democratic form of sexuality education contribute to the common good? After all, for example, scores of postmodernist scholars have argued that the modernist tradition, out of which liberalism emerged, has failed to deliver on its promises of liberty and equality for all. Instead, they argue, the liberal conception of democracy has, in fact, fostered economic, racial, ethnic, and gender oppression in the interests of a capitalist patriarchy. This is so, at least in part, because the principles of modernity have, according to Aronowitz and Giroux (1991), "been largely drawn from cultural scripts written by white males whose work is often privileged as a model of high culture" (p. 58) and that these principles represent "expressions of particular discourses embodying normative interests and legitimating historically specific relations of power" (p. 58). In sum, according to some postmodernists, the concept of liberal democracy is a ruse, employed by a privileged few in order to maintain power. [1]

Feminist and gay and lesbian scholars have quite correctly pointed out that the liberal modernist tradition has yet to bring them full liberty and equality. Indeed, they often argue, it is the structures of philosophical and political liberalism that have helped perpetuate, not combat, centuries of injustice, particularly as they pertain to gender and sexual orientation. For example, in philosophical terms, it is clear that political liberalism relies heavily on the desirability and presumed capacity of individuals to reason autonomously. As Rawls (1993) suggests,

> citizens think of themselves as free in three respects: first, as having the moral power to form, to revise, and rationally to pursue a conception of the good; second, as being self-authenticating sources of valid claims; and third, as capable of taking responsibility for their ends. Being free in these respects enables citizens to be both rationally and fully autonomous. (p. 72)

However, from the perspective of many feminists, "Throughout the history of western philosophy there is a demonstrable alignment between the ideals of autonomous reason and the ideals of masculinity" (Code, 1991, p. 117). Carol Gilligan (1982) argues that the preferred conceptualizations of moral reasoning, focussing on abstract autonomous reasoning, that have emerged from this philosophical tradition are suited to stereotypically masculine ways of sorting out moral dilemmas. This suggests, from some feminist perspectives, that as a philosophical tradition, liberalism has a limited potential to contribute to gender equality including its explicitly sexual elements.

James Sears (1992) asserts that,

> In the United States, the social construction of gender and sexuality (i.e., the transference of biological divisions of maleness and femaleness into social categories), the delegation of human roles and traits according to conceptions of femininity and masculinity, and the proscription of certain sexual activities rationalize a particular way of organizing society-patriarchy. (p. 144)

Here liberalism is seen as severely limited in its capacity to disrupt patriarchy. Because it generally restricts itself to the public domain and its institutions—remaining neutral in regard to the private realm of beliefs and social arrangements—political liberalism can do little to directly influence the social construction of gender and sexuality; it was never intended to do so.

Gay and lesbian critiques of liberalism have been argued along similar lines. Kitzinger (cited in Sears, 1992), in analyzing the social construction of lesbianism, contends that

> Our "inner selves"—the way we think and feel and how we define ourselves—are connected in an active and reciprocal way with the larger social and political structures and processes in the context of which they are constructed. It is for this reason that, as many radical and revolutionary movements and oppressed peoples have argued, "the personal is political." (p. 145)

Because it is not directly concerned with the personal, political liberalism circumvents the connection between the inner self and larger political structures. Thus, according to this view, the integrity of a given inner self, particulary the integrity of sexual minorities, cannot be protected from the hostility of those who, because of their ideology, disapprove of them. As Sullivan (1995) remarks,

> Indeed, the true liberal doesn't even pretend that his or her laws will solve the deepest problems of the human heart; liberalism is not, after

all, designed to counteract hostile feelings, but hostile *acts*. Liberalism at its best can stay aloof from the troubling problems of human sexuality, but still insist that a person not be fired for something utterly unrelated to his work, or evicted simply because he is homosexual, or subject to violence primarily because of his sexual orientation. (pp. 157-158)

These critiques reveal what are simultaneously both the strengths and weaknesses of political liberalism as the constitutive ethos of democratic society. In the private sphere, political liberalism cannot compel a bigot to mend his or her ways. Political liberalism cannot force a person to convert his or her hatred of homosexuals into love or to believe that women are not a subordinate sex. Political liberalism can only insist that in the public sphere, homosexuals and women must be accorded full equality, enjoying the same freedoms and rights as any other individual in society. But if this is a weakness it is also a strength. The strength of political liberalism is that by insisting that the private sphere be regulated by the principle of freedom of belief it allows oppressed groups such as women and homosexuals to enter their concerns, as persons deserving of freedom and equality, into public and political discourse. Thus, it is a positive attribute that political liberalism does not legislate the shape of an individual's moral beliefs other than to seek his or her respect for the overlapping consensus of a democratic society. While this limited scope of political liberalism, particularly as it applies to the private realm of individual moral belief, is clearly seen as a weakness by some, political liberalism has enjoyed some success in bringing greater social justice to the public realm. For example, although no one would argue that contemporary Western society is free of racism, the progressive struggles for racial equality that have occurred during the 20th century have had a considerable measure of success in terms of modifying public institutions for the purposes of reducing racial discrimination. In legislating against dis-crimination in hiring practices, housing, educational opportunity, etc., the struggle for racial equality was, and is, being fought on the basis of the fundamental liberal principles as they apply to the public sphere.

Similarly, with respect to discrimination based on gender and sexual orientation, political liberalism has been at least modestly successful in addressing these problems in the public sphere. For example, feminist attempts to use the structures of political liberalism in order to bring about changes in the public sphere have not been entirely futile. As Jagger (1982) notes,

> Primarily through the efforts of liberal feminists, the legal status of women in most of the industrialized nations has improved considerably in the last fifteen years. In the United States, many kinds of sex discrimination have been outlawed, new forms of discrimination, such as sexual harassment or denial of maternity leave, have been legally recognized, affirmative action programs are often required by law, the legal right to abortion has been established, although it remains under attack and in some areas the right to express one's sexual preference is legally protected. (p. 185)

In terms of sexual orientation, there can be no question that the legal status of homosexuals has improved significantly in recent years. And, as Sullivan (1995) suggests, "Without the liberal tradition, homosexuals—and most other minorities—would not enjoy the discussion which now ensnares them in Anglo-American politics, let alone the historically rare toleration that is now afforded them" (pp. 133-134).

None of this is intended to suggest that political liberalism is a cure-all for social injustice, capable of delivering full sexual equality to oppressed groups. The above examples do, however, auger well for a persuasive argument that a democratic philosophy of sexuality education, modeled on the overlapping consensus of political liberalism, provides a reasonable way of adjudicating the unreasonable amount of ideological bias in existing sexuality education in the schools.

Given our dependence on subjectively derived ideology to inform our thinking on sexuality, the higher order objective of a democratic philosophy of sexuality education in the public schools is not to cleanse young minds of sexual ideologies that we may disagree with. Rather, the higher order objective of a democratic philosophy of sexuality education is to provide a learning environment in which different beliefs are respected within the context of the overlapping consensus of democracy. Whereas the private sphere of individual beliefs about the nature and moral aspects of human sexuality is not legislatively prescribed by political liberalism, a democratic sexuality education does not attempt to dictate an individual's beliefs about sexuality. Where the public actions of individuals conflict with the basic freedoms of others, political liberalism seeks to legislate against discrimination. Conversely, a democratic sexuality education teaches respect for freedom of belief and respect for the overlapping consensus of reasonable doctrines in a democratic society. In sum, in learning about sexuality students are learning about democracy.

What the examples of gender and sexual orientation show is that while political liberalism cannot deliver a society in which everyone agrees with each other, it does appear to be equipped to provide an environment in which marginalized or oppressed groups can make a claim for equal rights in the public sphere of society. A liberal democracy is no longer democratic when these claims are silenced. While it can be argued with convincing evidence that neither women nor homosexuals have attained a position of equality, it would be much more difficult to argue that in contemporary public discourse their voices are not heard. In regard to this point, I have tried to show that one of the fundamental inadequacies of sexuality education in the schools is that due to ideological bias and political expediency, some of the many voices of differing perspectives on sexuality have been silenced.

Among the chief complaints against liberalism is that it represents a status quo with a tarnished history. However, the application of liberal democratic philosophy to sexuality education hardly represents the status quo. To the contrary, the modern history of sexuality education is, as I have tried to show, replete with examples of how the basic principles of democracy have often been flouted. Furthermore, it is difficult to imagine how, in its present incarnations, sexuality education can be inclusive of identity politics, the idea that our political beliefs and goals can and should be rooted in our identity based on sexual orientation, gender, etc., in its classroom discourse. Sexuality education, as it stands, is largely dominated by ideological perspectives that exclude identity politics. A democratic philosophy of sexuality education offers an opportunity for these voices to be expressed and to be subsequently either critically appropriated or rejected by individual students. A democratic philosophy of sexuality education represents a conscious effort to disrupt the status quo in teaching about sexuality in the schools. It is a philosophy aimed at teaching young people about sexuality in a way that is consistent with societal respect for the different sexual ideologies that co-exist in our culture and that is consistent with the basic values of society.

At its genesis, the debate about sexuality in general and sexuality education in particular is between the divergent ethics emerging from opposing sexual ideologies. An ethical theory which seeks to characterize or define the nature of human sexuality and to propose concrete criteria for judging sexual behaviour must, by its very nature, be rooted in a subjective sexual ideology. A pluralist democracy cannot remain true to itself if it allows its public institutions to favour or impose a particular sexual ideology on its people. Unfortunately, the public education system, perhaps the most potent of socializing agents, has often allowed itself to become a propagandizing platform for various sexual ideologies. In order to rectify this, we must turn to the principles of democracy itself to both remove the evil of ideological indoctrination in the schools and to educate young people about their rights and responsibilities in democratic society as they pertain to sexuality. In other words, sexuality education should not only be based upon a democratic philosophy of education in terms of its structure, but in content, sexuality education should be education that supports the ideals of democratic living.

For some time now our society has been engaged in a series of social, scientific, and moral reformations and counter-reformations related to sexuality. None of these transformations have been remotely close to being socially monolithic. As we have seen, with sexuality, our society is clearly divided along ideological lines. The lines of division are not always consistent or clear-cut: each ideology has its internal permutations that may, at times, overlap with other ideologies. On occasion, most seemingly opposed sexual ideologies are in agreement on specific issues. For example, nearly all the variants of both Restrictive and Permissive sexual ideology are currently united in their condemnation of sex between adults and children. However, more often than not, we can find little to agree on. Sexuality divides us as a culture, and these divisions are not trivial. They often relate to fundamental aspects of who we are and how we relate to each other, both as individuals and as a society. Thus, with so much at stake, our disagreements about sexuality are a serious concern.

In terms of sexuality education in our schools, the central question I have been trying to address is what do we do with this ideological diversity? Rather than affirming diversity, or at least tolerating it, as we might expect a democratic culture to do, our cultural discourse around sexuality has pitted one ideology against another in a battle for cultural supremacy. As this battle ebbs and flows, the result is a society and a people deeply ambivalent about a fundamental part of themselves. In the case of sexuality education this discord and ambivalence has paralysed the school in its ability to provide youth with a meaningful education about sexuality. Because our sexuality shoulders the burden of immense individual and social significance, a meaningful sexuality education is the right of all people. With beliefs about human sexuality currently in the grips of such widely divergent meaning

systems, political liberalism with its allegiance to the most basic and uncomplicated of democratic principles, is, at this stage of our development as a
culture, the most appropriate philosophical framework to broker these
differences. This may be particularly the case for public institutions such as
the school which must guard against choosing sides in social debates of this
kind.

In my research, I have found evidence of support for the type of
philosophy of education that I have proposed here. I have recently surveyed
several hundred parents in a community in Ontario, Canada on their
opinions and attitudes towards sexual health education in the schools
(McKay, 1996). Over 90% of the parents I surveyed believed that sexual
health education should be provided in the schools. Eighty percent of the
parents agreed with the statement "It is important for sexual health education programs to recognize and respect the different moral beliefs about
sexuality that may exist in the community." Just over 12% were unsure,
while only 7.3% disagreed with this statement. Over 70% of parents in this
survey expressed their approval for the topic "Moral Beliefs about Sexuality"
being included in school-based programs. In addition, a majority of parents
approved of the inclusion of such controversial topics as sexual orientation
and birth control. Recent replications of this study in other communities
have produced almost identical findings (Langille, Langille, Beazley, &
Doncaster, 1996; McKay et al., in press).

Although the public discourse on sexuality education has been characterized by intense ideological conflict, these surveys suggest the possibility
that most parents, who may not typically express their opinions about
sexuality education publicly, are less ideologically partisan in their beliefs
about the form and content of sexuality education in the schools than are
the vocal minority who dominate public discourse. The parents I surveyed
supported neither exclusive partiality or exclusive neutrality in the delivery
of sexuality education in the schools. They expressed support for sexuality
education in the schools that engages moral issues and respects moral
diversity related to sexuality. In these respects, I believe that these parents'
opinions are consistent with a democratic philosophy of sexuality education.
This is just one example of an increasing number of signs that the Western
tradition of allowing sexual ideology to dictate our lives is giving way to more
democratic ways of ordering social life. Not only is sexual pluralism becoming more evident, but the call for sexual democracy is growing louder. As
Nancy Rosenblum (1997) suggests, "Preoccupied with the formative effects

of sexuality on character and community, an increasing number of contemporary political theorists approach the legal regulation of sexual conduct and relations from the point of view of democratic principles" (p. 63).

The commitment to pluralism as one of the constituent values of a just society, at the very least, strongly implies that there is no single universally right or true account of the good person or good life. Since sexuality is so fundamentally imbued with personal and social significance, the affirmation of a pluralism of sexual ideologies, each with their own conceptions of the good person and the good life, is a necessary aspect of a society whose commitment to pluralism is genuine. In conceptualizing education for democracy, Mark Weinstein (1991) argues that

> what constitutes "good lives and good societies" is not fixed once and for all, but rather is open to reconsideration by individuals in a democracy, and is reflected in the process of mediating among competing views. Granting this, we can indicate what is preserved by conscious reproduction in democratic societies, that is, the deliberative process itself. (p. 11)

If we believe that an affirmation of pluralism and democracy are inseparable, as the liberal tradition holds, it follows that public institutions such as the school have an obligation to affirm and respect diverse sexual ideologies in their attempts to educate young people about sexuality. Brian Crittenden (1973) asks,

> If the members of a society have not yet reached an agreement on the content of what some consider an adequate range of beliefs and practices, how can any group in a democracy have authority to decide what this content should be, and to inculcate it through a public system of schooling? (p. 110)

Where ideological disputes about the form and content of school-based sexuality education exist, a democratic philosophy of sexuality education ought to prevail. Where such disputes do occur, policy makers who reject appeals to sexual ideology as foundations for promoting particular brands of sexuality education will be on firm ground to insist that democratic principles be respected in the creation and teaching of educational programs.

In articulating a democratic philosophy of sexuality education I have emphasized the distinction between lower order and higher order moral issues related to sexuality with the former pertaining to sexual ideology and the latter to democratic principles. In the end, to make this distinction is to ask that we be democratic citizens first and sexual ideologues second. No matter what sexual ideology we favour as individuals, school board trustees, court judges, or government representatives, it should behove us to employ and defend democratic principles in accomodating, balancing, and brokering the different ideological perspectives that clearly do exist in our society.

What are the concrete implications for every day life in Western society if we move from sexual ideology to democratic principles as the ethical framework through which public institutions and our culture as a whole address sexuality? The answer is that in a democratic sexual landscape where the freedom consciously to make knowledgable choices and respect for the rights of others to pursue their own conception of the good life are encouraged, we cannot say with certainty what sexual norms people will embrace. Although this prospect, laden with uncertainty, is troubling to many of us, the democratization of sexuality should be cause for optimism not fear.

There is no reason to believe, as some might suggest, that sexual norms existing within a society that has democratized sexuality will be predisposed to favouring decadent and unhealthy lifestyles and practices. In contrast to the status quo where individual and group norms related to sexuality often develop under the veils of ignorance, repression and shame, an emphasis on encouraging people both young and old to make fully informed critically appropriated choices about their sexuality lends itself not to anarchy, but, in many cases, to restraint. Empowered by an environment that encourages knowledge over ignorance and choice over imposed ideology people are more likely to think first and act second. We are constantly confronted in our society by examples of people who seem not to act in their own best interests when it comes to sexuality. But it is a simplistic and counterproductive logic to insist that the fact that emotion and impulse inevitably weigh on our sexual behaviour translates into a social and political imperative to place strict limits on our freedom to pursue our own conceptions of the good life related to sexuality. If the history of sexuality in Western culture teaches us anything it is that this strategy has persistently failed. If we can draw from the basic principles of democracy to develop an approach to sexuality that emphasizes the individual's rights to knowledge and critically appropriated choice combined with an emphasis on the equally important democratic responsibility to respect the rights of others, we can greatly enhance the potential for healthy sexuality among both persons and communities. Although it is in essence straightforward, such an approach will require a fundamental change in the way we look at sexuality in our culture. Yet, herein may lie our best chance to meaningfully confront the seemingly endemic anguish, deception, disease, and exploitation that is perpetually associated with sexuality.

There is also no good reason to believe that a society that democratizes sexuality will lose all of its basic traditions related to sexuality, some of which are both highly functional and ethically sound. It is clearly feared in some quarters that extending the freedom to choose one's own critically appropriated good life with respect to sexuality means, inevitably, the end of the traditional Western ideal of sexual monogamy as a major component of the nuclear family unit. This is a dubious prophecy. Despite the loosening grip of Restrictive sexual ideology, particularly in the 20th century, the hope for a permanent sexually monogamous marriage is a major life goal for most people today, including the younger generations. Even with the increased tendency for many people to delay marriage, perhaps a healthy phenomenon, and despite higher divorce rates, most people sooner or later settle into a marriage based, at least in part, on a sexual bond. It goes without saying, that this lifestyle can be fully consistent with a democratic approach to sexuality. Its popularity endures and society, even public institutions, can and will continue to support it. It is certainly conceivable that the prevalence of divorce and unhappy families can be reduced if those who choose monogamous marriage make that choice after thoughtful consideration of the other viable alternative conceptions of the good life rather than being forced into a uniform social structure for which they may not be suited. Such a transformation is not a disaster, it is simply the acknowledgement that the affirmation of a plurality of sexual ideologies increases the likelihood that an individual has the freedom to choose a conception of the good life with which she or he is comfortable and that is compatible with his or her desires and life goals. This cannot harm society, it can only better it.

Although the future is uncertain, as it always is in a democracy, we can be confident that if it is critical deliberation and respect for democratic principles that takes us forward, the future will be bright. The rigid imposition of sexual ideology, so long the modus operandi of Western culture, is the author of ignorance, unhappiness, and oppression. Extending the basic principles of democracy to sexuality can advance our culture in significant ways. Encouraging informed value judgements and personal choices combined with a tolerance and respect for those who think and act differently from ourselves is the marker of both a healthy sexuality and a genuinely free and democratic society.

Note

1. It is difficult to generalize about whether or not postmodernism is anti-democratic. According to Rosenau (1992, pp. 98-100) the more sceptical of postmodernists have been labelled as anti-democratic by virtue of their contention that the structures of the democratic political tradition are fallacious, whereas the more affirmative of postmodernists call for a "deepening of democracy." I have argued elsewhere (McKay, 1994) that to the extent that postmodernism rejects the validity of key modernist principles such as justice and equality, it has the potential to violate the fundamental precepts of democratic living, and therefore may provide an inadequate framework for the theory and practice of moral education.

Bibliography

Alan Guttmacher Institute. (1989). *Risk and responsibility: Teaching sex education in America's schools today*. New York: author.

Ajzenstat, J. and Gentiles, I. (1988). *Sex education in Canada: A survey of policies and programs*. Toronto: Human Life Research Institute.

Allgeier, E.R. (1983). Ideological barriers to contraception. In D. Byrne & W. Fisher (Eds.), *Adolescents, sex, and contraception* (pp. 171-206). Hillsdale, NJ: Lawrence Erlbaum.

Allgeier, A. & Allgeier, E.R. (1988). *Sexual interactions* (2nd Ed). Lexington, MA: D.C. Heath.

American School Health Association. (1991). *Sexuality education within comprehensive school health education*. Kent, OH: author.

Anchell, M. (1987). Sex education is harmful. In D. Bender & B. Leone (Eds.), *Teenage sexuality: Opposing viewpoints* (pp. 49-54). St. Paul, MN: Greenhaven Press.

Aronowitz, S. & Giroux, H. (1991). *Postmodern education: Politics, culture, and social sriticism*. Minneapolis, MN: University of Minnesota Press.

Barrett, M. (1994). Sexuality education in Canadian schools: An overview in 1994. *The Canadian Journal of Human Sexuality, 3*(3), 199-208.

Barrett, M., et al. (1995). Sexuality in Canada. In R. Francoeur. (Ed.), *International encyclopedia of sexuality*. New York: Continuum Press.

Bateson, M.C. & Goldsby, R. (1988). *Thinking AIDS: The social response to the biological threat*. New York: Addison Wesley.

Berger, P., & Luckmann, T. (1967). *The social construction of reality: A treatise in the sociology of knowledge*. New York: Doubleday.

Breasted, M. (1970). *Oh! Sex education!* New York: Praeger Publishers.

Brittion, P.O., de Mauro, D., & Gambrell, A. (1992). HIV/AIDS education: SIECUS study on HIV/AIDS education for schools finds states make progress but work remains. *SIECUS Report, 21*(1), 1-8.

Brown, S. & Eisenberg, L. (Eds.), (1995). *The best intentions: Unintended pregnancy and the well-being of children and families*. Washington, DC: National Academy Press.

Brownmiller, S. (1975). *Against our will: Men, women, and rape*. New York: Simon and Shuster.

Bruess, C., & Greenberg, J. (1994). *Sexuality education: Theory and practice*, (3rd ed.). Dubuque, IA: Brown and Benchmark.

Bruner, J. (1996). *The culture of education*. Cambridge, MA: Harvard University Press.

Bruner, J. (1990). *Acts of meaning*. Cambridge, MA: Harvard University Press.

Bullough, V. (1994). *Science in the bedroom: A history of sex research*. New York: Basic Books.

Buss, D. (1994). *The evolution of desire: Strategies of human mating*. New York: Basic Books.

Byers, S. (1991). Gender differences in the traditional sexual script: Fact or fiction? *SIECCAN Journal*, 6(4), 16-18.

Calamides, E. (1990). AIDS and STD education: What's really happening in our schools? *Journal of Sex Education and Therapy*, 16(1), 54-63.

Canadian Charter of Rights and Freedoms. (1987). Appendix B. In R. Ghosh & D. Ray. (Eds.), *Social change and education in Canada* (pp. 281-285). Toronto: Harcourt Brace Jovanovich.

Carballo, M. Tawil, O., & Holmes, K. (1991). Sexual behaviors: Temporal and cross-cultural trends. In J. Holmes, S.O. Aral, K.K. Holmes, & P.J. Hitchcock (Eds.), *Research issues in human behaviour and sexually transmitted diseases in the AIDS era* (pp. 122-139). Washington, DC: American Society for Microbiology.

Carlson, D. (1992). Ideological conflict and change in the sexuality curriculum. In J. Sears (Ed.), *Sexuality and the curriculum: The politics and practices of sexuality education* (pp. 34-58). New York: Teachers College Press.

Carmichael, D. (1994). Political ideologies and values. In T.C. Pocklington (Ed.), *Representative democracy: An introduction to politics and government* (pp. 57-92). Toronto: Harcourt, Brace and Company, Canada.

Carter, R. (1984). *Dimensions of moral education*. Toronto: University of Toronto Press.

Centers for Disease Control and Prevention. (1995). Trends in sexual risk behavior among high-school students - United States, 1990, 1991, and 1993. *Morbidity and Mortality Weekly Report*, 44(7), 121-123, 131, 132.

Christopher, S. and Roosa, M. (1990). An evaluation of an adolescent pregnancy prevention program: Is "just say no" enough? *Family Relations*, 69, 68-72.

Cladis, M. (1995). Education, virtue and democracy in the work of Emile Durkhiem. *Journal of Moral Education*, 24(1), 37-52.

Code, L. (1991). *What can she know?: Feminist theory and the construction of knowledge*. Ithaca, NY: Cornell University Press.

Connel, R.W. (1987). *Gender and power: Society, the person and sexual politics*. Cambridge, UK: Polity Press.

Crittenden, B. (1973). *Education and social ideals: A study in philosophy of education*. Toronto: Longman Canada.

Dafoe-Whitehead, B. (1994, October). The failure of sex education. *Atlantic Monthly*, 55-80.

Daley, D. (1997). Exclusive purpose: Abstinence-only proponents create federal entitlement in welfare reform. *SIECUS Report, 25*(4), 3-7.

Darling, C. & Mabe, A. (1989). Analyzing ethical issues in sexual relationships. *Journal of Sex Education and Therapy, 15*(4), 234-236.

Dawson, D. (1986). The effects of sex education on adolescent behavior. *Family Planning Perspectives, 8*(4), 162-170.

D'Emilio, J. & Freenman, E. (1988). *Intimate matters: A history of sexuality in America.* New York: Harper and Row.

Davis, M. (1983). *Smut: Erotic reality/obscene ideology.* Chicago: University of Chicago Press.

Davis, C. (1992). The state of sexual science: A look back at the 80s; a look ahead to the 90s. *Journal of Psychology and Human Sexuality, 5*(3), 9-18.

Dine Jacobs, C., & Wolf, E. (1995). School sexuality education and adolescent risk-taking behavior. *Journal of School Health, 65*(3), 91-95.

Diorio, J. (1982). Sex, love, and justice: A problem in moral education. *Educational Theory, 31*(3 and 4), 225-235.

Dollimore, J. (1991). *Sexual dissidence: Augustine to Wilde, Freud to Foucault.* Oxford: Clarendon Press.

Downs, A.C. & Scarborough Hillje, L. (1993). Historical and theoretical perspectives on adolescent sexuality: An overview. In T.P. Gullotta, G.R. Adams, & R. Montemayor (Eds.), *Adolescent sexuality* (pp. 1-34). Newbury Park, NJ: Sage Publications.

Duncan, A.R.C. (1979). Escapes from moral thinking. In D.B. Cochrane, C.M. Hamm, & A.C. Kazepides (Eds.), *The domain of moral education* (pp. 7-16). New York: Paulist Press.

Durkheim, E. (1961). *Moral education: A study in the theory and application of the sociology of education* (pp. 300-327). Translated by E.K. Wilson & H. Schnurer. New York: Free Press of Glencoe

Dworkin, A. (1987). *Intercourse.* New York: Free Press.

Earls, R., Fraser, J., & Sumpter, B. (1992). Sexuality education—in whose interest? An analysis of legislative, state agency, and local change arenas. In J. Sears (Ed.), *Sexuality and the curriculum: The politics and practices of sexuality education* (pp. 300-327). New York: Teachers College Press.

Ehrhardt, A. (1996). Editorial: Our view of adolescent sexuality —a focus on risk behavior without the developmental context. *American Journal of Public Health, 86*(11), 1523-1525.

Ehrhardt, A., Yingling, S., & Warne, P. (1991). Sexual behavior in the era of AIDS: What changed in the United States? *Annual Review of Sex Research, Volume II,* 25-48.

Eisenman, R. (1994). Conservative sexual values: Effects of an abstinence program on student attitudes. *Journal of Sex Education and Therapy, 20*(2), 75-78.

Ellis, A. (1990). Commentary on the status of sex research: An assessment of the sexual revolution. *Journal of Psychology and Human Sexuality, 3*(1), 5-18.

English, D., Hollibaugh, A., & Rubin, G. (1987). Talking sex: A conversation on sexuality and feminism. In Feminist Review (Eds.), *Sexuality: A reader* (pp. 63-81). London: Virago Press.

Fassinger, R. (1991). The hidden minority: Issues and challenges in working with lesbian women and gay men. *Counseling Psychologist, 19,* 157-176.

Fine, M. (1988). Sexuality, schooling and adolescent females: The missing discourse of desire. *Harvard Educational Review, 58*(1), 29-53.

Fisher, J.D. & Fisher, W.A. (1992). Changing AIDS-risk behavior. *Psychological Bulletin, 111*(3), 455-474.

Fisher, W. (1990). All together now: An integrated approach to preventing adolescent pregnancy and STD/HIV infection. *SIECUS Report, 18*(4), 1-11.

Flavel, J. (1985). *Cognitive Development* (2nd ed.). Englewood Cliffs, NJ: Prentice Hall.

Forrest, J., & Silverman, J. (1989). What public school teachers teach about preventing pregnancy, AIDS, and sexually transmitted diseases. *Family Planning Perspectives, 21*(2), 65-72.

Foucault, M. (1978). *The history of sexuality: An introduction, volume I.* New York: Vantage Books.

Francoeur, R., Perper, T., & Scherzer, N. (1991). *A descriptive dictionary and atlas of sexology.* New York: Greenwood Press.

Francoeur, R. (1987). Are traditional sex roles preferable to androgenous sex roles? In R. Francoeur (Ed.), *Taking sides: Clashing and controversial issues in human sexuality* (pp. 28-29). Guilford, CT: Dushkin Publishing.

Frankl, G. (1974). *The failure of the sexual revolution.* London: Nel Mentor.

Frayser, S. (1994). Defining normal childhood sexuality: An anthropological approach. *Annual Review of Sex Research, Volume V,* 173-217.

Freud, S. (1977). *On sexuality: Three essays on the theory of sexuality.* London: Penguin Books.

Freudenberg, N. (1989). Social and political obstacles to AIDS education, *SIECUS Report, 17*(6), 1-6.

Fromer, M.J. (1983). *Ethical issues in sexuality and reproduction.* St. Louis, MO: C.V. Mosby.

Frost, J. & Darroch-Forest, J. (1995). Understanding the impact of effective teenage pregnancy prevention programs. *Family Planning Perspectives, 27*(5), 188-195.

Fuchs Epstein, C. (1988). *Deceptive distinctions: Sex, gender, and the social order.* New Haven, CT: Yale University Press.

Furstenberg, F., Moore, K., & Peterson, J. (1985). Sex education and sexual experience among adolescents. *American Journal of Public Health, 75,* 1331-1332.

Gagnon, J. (1990). The explicit and implicit use of the scripting perspective in sex research. *Annual Review of Sex Research, Volume I,* 1-44.

Gagnon, J. & Simon, W. (1973). *Sexual conduct: The social sources of human sexuality.* Chicago: Aldine Publishing.

Gallup Poll. (1985). The 17th annual Gallup Poll of the public's attitudes towards the public schools. *Phi Delta Kappan, 67*(22), 35-47.

Gallup Poll. (1991). Sex in America. *Gallup Poll Monthly, 56,* 1-9, 71.

Geer, J. & O'Donohue, W. (Eds.), (1987). *Theories of human sexuality.* New York: Plenum Press.

Ghosh, R. & Ray, D. (1987). *Social change and education in Canada.* Toronto: Harcourt Brace Jovanovich, Canada.

Giddens, A. (1987). *Sociology: A brief but critical introduction,* (2nd ed.). New York: Harcourt Brace Jovanovich.

Gilder, G. (1987). Sexual suicide. In R. Francoeur, (Ed.), *Taking sides: Clashing views on controversial issues in human sexuality* (pp. 30-37). Guilford, CT: Dushkin Publishing.

Gilligan, C. (1982). *In a different voice: Psychological theory and women's development.* Cambridge: Harvard University Press.

Giroux, H. and McLaren, P. (1992). Forward: Education for democracy. In J. Goodman, *Elementary schooling for critical democracy* (pp. xi-xviii). New York: State University of New York Press.

Goodman, J. (1992). *Elementary schooling for critical democracy.* New York: State University of New York Press.

Goodson, P. & Edmunson, E. (1994). The problematic promotion of abstinence: An overview of Sex Respect. *Journal of School Health, 65*(4), 205-210.

Greely, A. (1988). *Sexual intimacy: Love and play.* New York: Warner Books.

Greenberg, D. (1988). *The construction of homosexuality.* Chicago: University of Chicago Press.

Grunseit, A. and Kippax, S. (1993). *Effects of sex education on young people's sexual behavior.* Geneva: World Health Organization.

Guindon, A. (1986). *The sexual creators: An ethical proposal for concerned christians.* Lanham: University Press of America.

Guttmacher, S. (1997). Condom availability in New York City public high schools: Relationships to condom use and sexual behavior. *American Journal of Public Health, 87*(9), 1427-1433.

Guttman, A. (1987). *Democratic education.* Princeton, NJ: Princeton University Press.

Habermas, J. (1990). *Moral consciousness and communicative action.* Cambridge, MA: MIT Press.

Haffner, D. & De Mauro, D. (1991). *Winning the battle: Developing support for sexuality and HIV/AIDS education.* New York: SIECUS.

Haffner, D. (1992). Sexuality education in policy and practice. In J. Sears (Ed.), *Sexuality and the curriculum: The politics and practices of sexuality education* (pp. vii-viii). New York: Teachers College Press.

Hatfield, E., & Rapson, R. (1993). Historical and cross-cultural perspectives on passionate love and sexual desire. *Annual Review of Sex Research, Volume IV,* 67-98.

Haydon, G. (1995). Thick or thin? The cognitive content of moral education in a plural democracy. *Journal of Moral Education, 24*(1), 53-64.

Health Canada. (1994). *Canadian guidelines for sexual health education.* Ottawa: Ministry of National Health and Welfare.

Henslin, J. (1978). "Toward the sociology of sex." In J. Henslin & E. Sagarin (Eds.), *The sociology of sex* (pp. 1-25). New York: Schocken Books.

Hentoff, N. (1992). *Free speech for me - but not for thee: How the American left and right relentlessly censor each other.* New York: HarperCollins Publishers.

Hersh, R., Miller, J., & Fielding, G. (1980). *Models of moral education: An appraisal.* New York: Longman.

Hoffer, E. (1951). *The true believer: Thoughts on the nature of mass movements.* New York: Harper and Row.

Hoffman, S. (1995). Dreams of a just world. *The New York Review of Books, 42*(17), 52-56.

Holtzman, D. & Greene, B. (1992). HIV education and health education in the United States: A national survey of local health districts and practices. *Journal of School Health, 62*(9), 421-427.

Holtzman, D. et al. (1995). Trends in risk behaviors among U.S. high school students, 1989-1991. *AIDS Education and Prevention, 7*(3), 265-277.

Howard, M. & McCabe, J. (1990). Helping teenagers postpone sexual involvement. *Family Planning Perspectives, 22*(1), 21-26.

Irvine, J. (1990). *Disorders of desire: Sex and gender in modern American sexology.* Philadelphia: Temple University Press.

Jagger, A. (1983). *Feminist politics and human nature.* Sussex: Harvester Press.

Janus, S. & Janus, C. (1993). *The Janus report on sexual behavior.* New York: John Wiley and Sons, Inc.

Jeffreys, S. (1990). *Anticlimax: A feminist perspective on the sexual revolution.* New York: New York University Press.

Joffe, C. (1993). Sexual politics and the teenage pregnancy prevention worker in the United States. In A. Lawson & D. Rhode (Eds.), *The politics of pregnancy: Adolescent sexuality and public policy* (pp. 284-300). New Haven, CT: Yale University Press.

Johnstone, R. (1975). *Religion and society in interaction: The sociology of religion.* Englewood Cliffs, NJ: Prentice-Hall.

Jones, E.F. & Forrest, J. (1992). Contraceptive failure rates based on the 1988 NSFG. *Family Planning Perspectives, 24,* 21-29.

Jorgensen, S., Potts, V., & Camp, B. (1993). Project taking charge: Six month follow-up of a pregnancy prevention program for early adolescents. *Family Relations, 42,* 401-406.

Kaltsounis, T. (1994). Democracy's challenge as the foundation for social studies. *Theory and Research in Social Education, 22*(2), 176-193.

Kantor, L. (1993). Scared chaste? Fear-based educational curricula. *SIECUS Report, 21*(2), 1-15.

Kantor, L. (1994). Attacks on public school sexuality education programs: 1993-19994 school year. *SIECUS Report, 22*(6), 11-16.

Kardiner, A. (1955). *Sex and morality*. London: Routledge and Kegan Paul Ltd.

Karmel, L. (1970). Sex education, no; sex information, yes. *Phi Delta Kappan, 52,* 95-96.

Kelley, K. (1983). Adolescent sexuality: The first lessons. In D. Byrne & W. Fisher (Eds.), *Adolescents, sex, and contraception* (pp. 125-142). Hillsdale, NJ: Lawrence Erlbaum Associates.

Kelly, J. (1995). *Changing HIV risk behavior: Practical strategies*. New York: The Gilford Press.

Kelly, T. (1986). Discussing controversial issues: four perspectives on the teacher's role. *Theory and Research in Social Education, 14*(7), 113-138.

Kilpatrick, W. (1993). *Why Johnny can't tell right from wrong and what we can do about it*. New York: Touchstone Books.

King, A., Beazley, R., Warren, W., Hawkins, C., Robertson, A. & Radford, J. (1988). *Canada youth and AIDS study*. Kingston, ON: Social Program Evaluation Group, Queen's University.

Kirby, D. (1984). *Sexuality education: An evaluation of programs and their effects*. Santa Cruz, CA: Network Publications.

Kirby, D. (1992). School-based programs to reduce sexual risk-taking behaviors. *Journal of School Health, 62,* 280-287.

Kirby, D., et al. (1994). School-based programs to reduce sexual risk behaviors: A review of effectiveness. *Public Health Reports, 109*(3), 339-360.

Kitzinger, C. (1996). Speaking of oppression: Psychology, politics, and the language of power. In E. Rothblum & L. Bond (Eds.), *Preventing hetrosexism and homophobia* (pp. 3-18). Thousand Oaks, CA: Sage Publications.

Klassen, A., Williams, C., & Levitt, E. (1989). *Sex and morality in the U.S.: An empirical enquiry under the auspices of The Kinsey Institute*. Middletown, CT: Wesleyan University Press.

Kohlberg, L. (1974). Moral stages and sex education. In M. Calderone (Ed.), *Sexuality and human values: The personal dimension of sexual experience* (pp. 111-122). New York: Association Press.

Kohlberg, L. (1981). *The philosophy of moral development: Moral stages and the idea of justice, volume 1*. San Francisco: Harper and Row.

Kohlberg, L. (1984). *The psychology of moral development: Moral stages and the life cycle, volume 2*. San Francisco: Harper and Row.

Kosnick, A., Carroll, W., Cunningham, A., Modras, R., & Schulte, J. (1977). *Human sexuality: New directions in American Catholic thought, a study commissioned by the Catholic Theological Society of America*. New York: Paulist Press.

Ku, L., Sonnenstein, F., & Pleck, H. (1992). The association of AIDS education with sexual behavior and condom use among teenage men. *Family Planning Perspectives, 24* (2), 100-106.

Kuhn, T. (1970). *The Structure of Scientific Revolutions*. (2nd ed.). Chicago: University of Chicago Press.

LaCursia, N., Beyer, C., & Ogletree, R. (1994). The importance of a philosophy in sexuality education. *Family Life Educator, 13*(1), 4-9.

LaHaye, T. (1987). Sex education belongs in the home. In D. Bender & B. Leone (Eds.), *Teenage sexuality: Opposing view points* (pp. 55-60). St. Paul, MN: Greenhaven Press.

Langille, D., Langille, D., Beazley, R., & Doncaster, H. (1996). *Amherst parents' attitudes towards school-based sexual health education.* Amherst, NS: Amherst Initiative For Healthy Adolescent Sexuality.

Larrian, J. (1979). *The concept of ideology.* London: Hutchinson.

Laumann, E.O., Gagnon, J., Michael, R., & Michaels, S. (1994). *The social organization of sexuality: Sexual practices in the United States.* Chicago: University of Chicago Press.

Lawlor, W. & Purcell, L. (1989). Values and opinions about sex education among Montreal-area English secondary school students. *SIECCAN Journal, 4*(2), 26-34.

Lawlor, W., Morris, R., McKay, A., Purcell, L., & Comeau, L. (1990). Human sexuality education and the search for values. *SIECUS Report, 18*(6), 4-14.

Lenskyj, H. (1990). Beyond plumbing and prevention: Feminist approaches to sex education. *Gender and Education, 2*(2), 217-230.

Lickona, T. (1991). *Educating for character: How our schools can teach respect and responsibility.* New York: Bantam Books.

Lohrman, D. (1987). Exposing sexual exploitation through values voting. *Journal of School Health, 57*(6), 240-241.

Louis Harris Associates. (1988). *Public attitudes toward teenage pregnancy, sex education, and birth control.* New York: Planned Parenthood Federation of America.

Mackie, M. (1987). *Constructing women and men: Gender socialization.* Toronto: Holt, Rinehart, and Winston.

MacKinnon, C. (1987). A feminist/political approach: Pleasure under the patriarchy. In J.H. Geer & W.T. O'Donohue (Eds.), *Theories of human sexuality* (pp. 65-90). New York: Plenum Press.

MacKinnon, C. (1982). Feminism, marxism, method, and the state: An agenda for theory. *Signs, 7,* 519-544.

Manitoba Education and Training. (1990). *Family life education, grade 9: An optional health education unit.* Winnipeg, MB: Ministry of Education and Training.

Manley-Casimir, M. & Sussel, T. (1987). The "chartered" path: The new rights reality in Canadian society. In R. Ghosh & D. Ray (Eds.), *Social change and education in Canada* (pp. 170-183). Toronto: Harcourt Brace Johanovich.

Marcuse, H. (1966). *Eros and civilization: A philosophical inquiry into Freud.* Boston: Beacon.

Marsiglio, W. (1993). Attitudes toward homosexual activity and gays as friends: A national survey of heterosexual 15-to-19-year-old males. *The Journal of Sex Research, 30*(1), 12-17.

Marsiglio, W. & Mott, F. (1986). The impact of sex education on sexual activity, contraceptive use and premarital pregnancy among American teenagers. *Family Planning Perspectives, 18*(4), 151-162.

Marsmen, J. & Herold, E. (1986). Attitudes toward sex education and values in sex education. *Family Relations, 35,* 357-361.

Martin, D. (1988). The stigmatization of the gay and lesbian adolescent. In M. Schneider, *Often invisable: Counselling gay & lesbian youth* (pp. 59-69). Toronto: Central Toronto Youth Services.

Mass, L. (1990). *Dialogues of the sexual revolution, Volume 1: Homosexuality and sexuality.* New York: The Haworth Press.

Mauldon, J. & Luker, K. (1996). The effects of contraceptive education on method use at first intercourse. *Family Planning Perspectives, 28*(1), 19-24.

McCormick, N. (1994). *Sexual salvation: Affirming women's sexual rights and pleasures.* Westport, CT: Praeger.

McKay, A. (1993). Research supports broadly based sex education. *Canadian Journal of Human Sexuality, 2*(2), 89-98.

McKay, A. (1994). The implications of postmodernism for moral education. *The McGill Journal of Education, 29*(1), 31-44.

McKay, A. & Barrett, M. (1995). The Canadian guidelines for sexual health education: Issues related to interpretation and implementation. *Canadian Journal of Human Sexuality, 4*(1), 61-73.

McKay, A. (1996). Rural parents attitudes toward school-based sexual health education. *Canadian Journal of Human Sexuality, 5*(1), 15-24.

McKay, A. & Holowaty, P. (1997). Sexual health education: A study of adolescents' opinions, self-perceived needs, and current and preferred sources of information. *Canadian Journal of Human Sexuality, 6*(1), 29-38.

Medical Institute for Sexual Health. (1993). Directive abstinence sex education: What is it? Why is it vital? *Sexual Health Update, 1*(3), 1-2.

Mellanby, A., Phelps, F., Crichton, N., & Tripp, J. (1995). School sex education: An experimental programme with educational and medical benefit. *British Medical Journal, 311,* 414-417.

Meredith, P. (1989). *Sex education: Political issues in Britain and Europe.* New York: Routledge.

Michael, R., Gagnon, J., Laumann, E., & Kolata, G. (1994). *Sex in America: A definitive survey.* New York: Little, Brown and Company.

Michaels, S. (1997). The prevalence of homosexuality in the United States. In R.P. Cabaj & T.S. Stein (Eds.), *Textbook of homosexuality and mental health* (pp. 43-64). Washington, DC: American Psychiatric Press.

Middleman, A.B. (1996, September). Public policy regarding adolescent sexuality in a truly liberal state. *Politics and the Life Sciences,* 305-307.

Mitchell, A. (1993, Feb. 18). Faith, hope, and chastity. *Globe and Mail,* A-1, A-10.

Mitchell, A. & Laghi, B. (1997, November 20). Calgary board bans two books. *Globe and Mail,* A-14.

Money, J. & Tucker, P. (1975). *Sexual signatures: On being a man or a woman.* Boston: Little, Brown and Company.

Money, J. (1985). *The destroying angel.* Buffalo: Prometheus Books.

Money, J. (1991). Sexology and/or sexosophy: The split between sexual researchers and reformers in history and practice. *SIECUS Report, 19*(3), 1-4.

Moon, J.D. (1993). *Constructing community: Moral pluralism and tragic conflicts.* Princeton, NJ: Princeton University Press.

Morris, R. (1993). Teaching values in sexuality education: From value-freedom to neutrality and beyond. *Canadian Journal of Human Sexuality, 2*(2), 71-79.

Morris, R. (1994). *Values in sexuality education: A philosophical study.* Lanham, MD: University Press of America.

Morrison, E. & Price, M. (1974). *Values in sexuality: A new approach to sex education.* New York: Hart Publishing.

Mosher, D. (1989). The threat to sexual freedom: Moralistic intolerance instills a spiral of silence. *The Journal of Sex Research, 26*(4), 492-509.

Mosher, D. (1991). Ideological predispositions: Rhetoric in sexual science, sexual politics, and sexual morality. *Journal of Psychology and Human Sexuality, 4*(4), 7-29.

Mosher, R., Kenny, R., & Garrod, A. (1994). *Preparing for citizenship: Teaching youth to live democratically.* Westport, CT: Praeger.

National Guidelines Taskforce. (1991). *Guidelines for comprehensive sexuality education, kindergarten - 12th Grade.* New York: SIECUS.

Naus, J. & Theis, J. (1991). The construction of sexuality: Implications for sex education and sex therapy. *SIECCAN Journal, 6*(4), 19-24.

Nelson, K.L. (1996). The conflict over sexuality education: Interviews with participants on both sides of the debate. *SIECUS Report, 24*(6), 12-16.

Nelson, J. (1988). *The intimate connection: Male sexuality, masculine spirituality.* Philadelphia: The Westminster Press.

Neutens, J. (1992). Sexuality education in comprehensive school health programs: Escaping the "moral smog." *Journal of School Health, 62*(2), 74-75.

Neutens, J. (1994). Sexuality education: A kaleidoscope of interpretations. In J. Drolet & K. Clark (Eds.), *The sexuality education challenge: Promoting healthy sexuality in young people* (pp. 29-46). Santa Cruz, CA: ETR Associates.

New Brunswick Department of Education. (1989). *Health and physical education 110: Addendum - AIDS education.* Fredericton, NB: author.

Okin, S.M. (1997). Sexual orientation and gender: Dichotomizing differences. In D.M. Estland & M.C. Nussbaum (Eds.), *Sex, preference, and family: Essays on law and nature* (pp. 44-62). New York: Oxford University Press.

Olsen, J. et al. (1992). Student evaluation of sex education programs advocating abstinence. *Adolescence, 7*, 369-380.

Ornstein, M. (1989). *AIDS in Canada: Knowledge, behaviour, and attitudes of adults.* Toronto: Institute for Social Research, York University.

Ozmon, H. & Craver, S. (1986). *Philosophical foundations of education, third edition.* Toronto: Merrill Publishing Company.

Pagels, E. (1988). *Adam, Eve, and the serpent.* New York: Vintage Books.

Pearson, A. (1992). Teacher education in a democracy. *Educational Philosophy and Theory, 24*(1), 83-92.

P.E.I. Department of Education. (1988). *Senior high (grade 10) family life education.* Charlottetown, PEI: author.

Phariss, T. (1997). Public schools: A battleground in the cultural war. In W. Swan (Ed.), *Gay/lesbian/bisexual/transgender public policy issues: A citizen's and administrator's guide to the new cultural struggle* (pp. 75-90). New York: The Howorth Press.

Philips, L., & Fine, M. (1992). Whats "left" in sexuality education. In J. Sears (Ed.), *Sexuality and the curriculum: The politics and practices of sexuality education* (pp. 242-250). New York: Teachers College Press.

Pollis, C. (1985). Value judgements and world views in sexuality education. *Family Relations, 34,* 285-290.

Posner, R. (1992). *Sex and reason.* Cambridge, MA: Harvard University Press.

Potter, S. & Roach, N. (1990). *Sexuality, commitment & family: Senior high student text.* Spokane, WA: Teen-Aid, Inc.

Progoff, I. (1963). *The symbolic and the real: A new psychological approach to the fuller experience of personal existence.* New York: McGraw Hill Publishers.

Rademakers, R. (1995). Preventing adolescent pregnancy: Model programs and evaluations. *Archives of Sexual Behavior, 24*(3), 358-360.

Raths, L., Harmin, M. and Simon, S. (1978). *Values and teaching: Working with values in the classroom.* (2nd Ed). Columbus, OH: Charles E. Merrill.

Rawls, J. (1971). *A theory of justice.* Cambridge, MA: Belknap.

Rawls, J. (1993). *Political liberalism.* New York: Columbia University Press.

Reich, W. (1971). *The inversion of compulsory sexual morality.* New York: Farrar, Straus, and Giroux.

Rest, J. (1984). The major components of morality. In W. Kurtines & J. Gewirtz (Eds.), *Morality, moral behavior, and moral development.* New York: John Wiley and Sons.

Reimer, J., Paolitto, D., & Hersh, R. (1983). *Promoting moral growth: From Piaget to Kohlberg.* (2nd ed.). New York: Longman Inc.

Reiss, M. (1997). Teaching about homosexuality and heterosexuality. *Journal of Moral Education, 26*(3), 343-352.

Reiss, I. (1993). The future of sex research and the meaning of science. *The Journal of Sex Research, 30*(1), 3-11.

Reiss, I. (1990). *An end to shame: Shaping our next sexual revolution.* Buffalo: Prometheus Books.

Rhode, D. (1993). Adolescent pregnancy and public policy. In A. Lawson & D. Rhode (Eds.), *The politics of pregnancy: Adolescent sexuality and public policy* (pp.301-306). New Haven, CT: Yale University Press.

Rienzo, B. (1989). The politics of sexuality education. *Journal of Sex Education and Therapy, 15*(3), 163-174.

Riesman, J. & Eichel, E. (1990). *Kinsey, sex and Fraud: The indoctrination of a people*. Lafayette, LA: Huntington House.

Robinson, P. (1976). *The modernization of sex: Havelock Ellis, Alfred Kinsey, William Masters and Virginia Johnson*. Ithaca, NY: Cornell University Press.

Roosa, M. & Christopher, S. (1990). Evaluation of an abstinence-only adolescent pregnancy prevention program: A replication. *Family Relations, 39*, 363-367.

Rosenau, P.M. (1992). *Post-modernism and the social sciences: Insights, inroads, and intrusions*. Princeton: Princeton University Press.

Rosenblum, N.L. (1997). Democratic sex: Reynolds v. U.S., sexual relations, and community. In D.M. Estlund & M.A. Nussbaum (Eds.), *Sex, preference, and family: Essays on law and nature* (pp. 63-85). New York: Oxford University Press.

Ross, S. & Kantor, L. (1995). Trends in opposition to comprehensive sexuality education in public schools: 1994-95 school year. *SIECUS Report, 23*(6), 9-15.

Rubin, G. (1984). Thinking sex: Notes for a radical theory of the politics of sexuality. In C. Vance (Ed.), *Pleasure and danger: Exploring female sexuality*. Boston: Routledge and Kegan Paul.

Rubin, I. (1970). The sex educator and moral values. In SIECUS (Eds.), *Sexuality and man*. New York: Charles Scribner and Sons.

Ruenzel, D. (1993). Going too far. *Teacher Magazine, 5*(3), 22-27.

Ruse, M. *Homosexuality: A philosophical inquiry*. New York: Basil Blackwell Ltd.

Sanderson, C. & Wilson, S. (1991). Desperately seeking abstinence: A critique of the Teen-Aid curricula for sexuality education. *SIECUS Report, 19*(5), 28-29.

Sapon-Shevin, M. & Goodman, J. (1992). Learning to be the opposite sex: Sexuality education and sexual scripting in early adolescence. In J. Sears (Ed.), *Sexuality and the curriculum: The politics and practices of sexuality education* (pp. 89-105). New York: Teachers College Press.

Saul, J.R. (1993). *Voltaire's bastard's: The dictatorship of reason in the west*. Toronto: Penguin Books.

Scales, P. & Roper, M. (1994). Challenges to sexuality education in the schools. In J. Drolet & K. Clark (Eds.), *The sexuality education challenge: Promoting healthy sexuality in young people* (pp. 69-92). Santa Cruz, CA: ETR Associates.

Schlafly, P. (1983). "What's wrong with sex education?" In B. Leone & T. O'Neill (Eds.), *Sexual values: Opposing viewpoints* (pp. 45-49). St. Paul, MN: Greenhaven Press.

Schur, E. (1988). *The Americanization of sex*. Philadelphia: Temple University Press.

Sears, J. (1992). Dilemmas and possibilities of sexuality education: Reproducing the body politic. In J. Sears (Ed.), *Sexuality and the curriculum: The politics and practices of sexuality education* (pp. 7-33). New York: Teachers College Press.

Sears, J. (1992). The impact of culture and ideology on the construction of gender and sexual identities: Developing a critically based sexuality curriculum. In J. Sears (Ed.), *Sexuality and the curriculum: The politics and practices of sexuality education* (pp. 139-156). New York: Teachers College Press.

Sedway, M. (1992). Fear right takes aim at sexuality education. *SIECUS Report,* 20(3), 13-19.

Seidman, S. (1992). *Emabattled eros: Sexual politics and ethics in contemporary America.* New York: Routledge.

Sellors, D., McGraw, S., & Mickinlay, J. (1994). Does the promotion and distribution of condoms increase teen sexual activity? Evidence from an HIV prevention program for latino youth. *American Journal of Public Health, 84,* 1952-1957.

Sethna, C. (1994). Nature, natural, naturalist: Nature study and the teaching of biological reproduction in Ontario, 1900-1930. *Canadian Journal of Human Sexuality, 3*(3), 191-198.

Shapiro, R. & Francoeur, R. (1987). We should recognize current alternatives to traditional monogamy? In R. Francoeur (Ed.), *Taking sides: Clashing and controversial issues in human sexuality* (pp. 88-96). Guilford, CT: Dushkin Publishing.

SIECUS. (1993). SIECUS fact sheet #4 on comprehensive sexuality education: The far right and fear-based abstinence-only programs. *SIECUS Report, 21*(2), 16-18.

Simon, W. (1994). Deviance as history: The future of perversion. *Archives of Sexual Behavior, 23*(1), 1-20.

Simon, W. (1989). Commentary on the status of sex research: The postmodernization of sex. *Journal of Psychology and Human Sexuality, 2*(1), 9-37.

Smart, C. (1995). *Law, crime and sexuality: Essays in feminism.* London: Sage Publications.

Smith, T. (1994). Attitudes toward sexual permissiveness: Trends, correlates, and behavioral connections. In A. Rossi (Ed.), *Sexuality across the life course* (pp. 63-94). Chicago: University of Chicago Press.

Spindel, B. & Duby, B. (1994) "Attacks on the freedom to learn: People for the American way's report on school censorship." *SIECUS Report, 23*(1).

Spinks, S. (1963). *Psychology and religion: An introduction to contemporary views.* London: Methuen and Co.

Stanton, D. (1992). The subject of sexuality. In D. Stanton (Ed.), *Discourse of sexuality: From Aristotle to AIDS.* Ann Arbor, MI: University of Michigan Press.

Steedman, M. (1987). Who's on top: Heterosexual practices and male dominance during the sex act. In H. Buchbinder & V. Burstyn (Eds.), *Who's on top: The politics of heterosexuality.* Toronto: Garamond Press.

Strong, B. & DeVault, C. (1994). *Human sexuality.* Toronto: Mayfield Publishing Company.

Stout, W. & Rivara, F. (1989). Schools and sex education: Does it work? *Pediatrics, 83,* 375-379.

Struening, K. (1995). Privacy and sexuality in a society divided over moral culture. *Political Research Quarterly, 49*(3), 479-504.

Sullivan, A. (1995). _Virtually normal: An argument about homosexuality._ New York: Alfred A. Knopf.

Swan, W. (1997). The agenda for justice. In W. Swan (Ed.), _Gay/lesbian/bisexaul/transgender public policy issues: A citizen's and administrator's guide to the new cultural struggle_ (pp. 123-129). New York: The Haworth Press.

Symons, D. (1979). _The evolution of human sexuality._ New York: Oxford University Press.

Szasz, T. (1980). _Sex by prescription._ New York: Doubleday.

Szirom, T. (1988). _Teaching gender? Sex education and sexual stereotypes._ Boston: Allen and Unwin.

Thompson, R. (1994). Moral rhetoric and public health pragmatism: The recent politics of sex education. _Feminist Review, 48,_ 40-60.

Thompson, J. (1984). _Studies in the theory of ideology._ Berkeley, CA: University of California Press.

Tiefer, L. (1995). _Sex is not a natural act and other essays._ San Francisco: Westview Press.

Troiden, R. & Platt, J. (1987). Does sexual ideology correlate with level of sexual experience? Assessing the construct validity of the SAS. _Journal of Sex Research, 23_(2), 256-260.

Trudell, B. (1992). "Inside a ninth-grade sexuality classroom: The process of knowledge construction." In J. Sears (Ed.), _Sexuality and the curriculum: The Politics and practices of sexuality education_ (pp. 203-225). New York: Teachers College Press.

Trudell, B. & Whatley, M. (1991). Sex respect: A problematic public school sexuality curriculum. _Journal of Sex Education and Therapy, 17_(2), 125-140.

Udry, J.R. (1993). The politics of sex research. _The Journal of Sex Research, 30_(2), 103-110.

Vance, C. (1984). _Pleasure and danger: Exploring female sexualtiy._ Boston: Routledge and Kegan Paul.

Verby, C. & Herold, E. (1992). Parents and AIDS education. _AIDS Education and Prevention, 4,_ 187-198.

Verene, D.P. (1972). _Sexual love and western morality: A philosophical anthology._ New York: Harper Torchbooks.

Vincent, M. & Pfefferkarn, L. (1994). The affective dimension: A prerequisite for effective sexuality education. In J. Drolet & K. Clark (Eds.) _The sexuality education challenge: Promoting healthy sexuality in young people_ (pp. 235-253). Santa Cruz, CA: ETR Associates.

Ward, O. (1971). The new morality: A christian perspective. In D. Grummon & A. Barclay (Eds.), _Sexuality: A search for perspective_ (pp. 204-212). New York: Van Nostrund Reinhold Company.

Weed, S. & Jensen, L. (1993). A second year evaluation of three abstinence sex education programs. _Journal of Research and Development in Education, 26,_ 92-96.

Weeks, J. (1985). *Sexuality and its discontents: Meanings, myths, and modern sexualities*. London: Routledge and Kegan Paul.

Weeks, J. (1986). *Sexuality*. New York: Tavistock Publications.

Weeks, J. (1992). Values in an age of uncertainty. In D. Stanton (Ed.), *Discourses of sexuality: From Aristole to AIDS* (pp. 389-411). Ann Arbor, MI: The University of Michigan Press.

Weeks, J. (1995). *Invented moralities: Sexual values in an age of uncertainty*. New York: Columbia University Press.

Weinstein, M. (1991). Critical thinking and education for democracy. *Educational Philosophy and Theory, 23*(3), 9-29.

Welle, H., Russel, R., & Kittleson, M. (1995). Philosophical trends in health education: Implications for the 21st century. *Journal of Health Education, 26*(6), 326-332.

Wellings, K. et al. (1995). Provision of sex education and early sexual experience: The relation examined. *British Medical Journal, 311*, 251-271.

Welsherimer, K., & Harris, S. (1994). A survey of rural parents attitudes toward sexuality education. *The Journal of School Health, 64*(9), 347-352.

Whatley, M. (1987). Biological determinism and gender issues in sexuality education. *Journal of Sex Education and Therapy, 13*(2), 26-29.

Whatley, M. (1988). Raging hormones and powerful cars: The construction of men's sexuality in school sex education and popular adolescent films. *Journal of Education, 170*(3), 100-121.

Whatley, M. (1992). Whose sexuality is it anyway? In J. Sears (Ed.), *Sexuality and the curriculum: The politics and practices of sexuality education* (pp. 78-84). New York: Teachers College Press.

Whatley, M. & Trudell, B. (1993). Teen-Aid: Another problematic sexuality curriculum. *Journal of Sex Education and Therapy, 19*(4), 251-271.

Wright, R. (1994). *The moral animal, why we are the way we are: The new science of evolutionary psychology*. New York: Vintage Books.

Yarber, W. (1992). While we stood by: The limiting of sexual information to our youth. *Journal of Health Education, 23*(6), 326-335.

Yarber, W. (1993). *STDs and AIDS: A guide for today's young adults, student manual*. Reston, VA: American Alliance for Health, Physical Education and Dance.

Yarber, W. (1994). Past, present and future perspectives on sexuality education. In J. Drolet & K. Clark (Eds.), *The sexuality education challenge: Promoting healthy sexuality in young people* (pp. 3-28). Santa Cruz, CA: ETR Associates.

Zabin, L. & Hayward, S. (1993). *Adolescent sexual behavior and childbearing*. Newbury Park, CA: Sage Publications.

Zelnik, M. & Kim, Y. (1982). Sex education and its association with teenage sexual activity, pregnancy, and contraceptive use. *Family Planning Perspectives, 16*, 117-126.

Index

—··—··